WHEN I'M GONE

Practical Notes for Those You Leave Behind

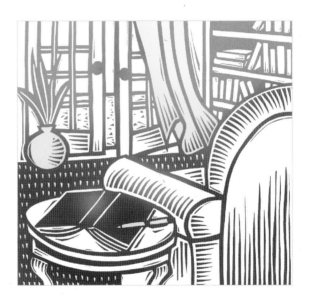

Kathleen Fraser

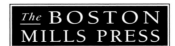
The BOSTON
MILLS PRESS

A Boston Mills Press Book

Copyright © 2009 Kathleen Fraser

Thirteenth printing, 2016

First published by Boston Mills Press, 2009

In Canada:
Distributed by Firefly Books Ltd.
50 Staples Avenue, Unit 1
Richmond Hill, Ontario, Canada L4B 0A7

In the United States:
Distributed by Firefly Books (U.S.) Inc.
P.O. Box 1338, Ellicott Station
Buffalo, New York 14205

Library and Archives Canada Cataloguing in Publication

Fraser, Kathleen, 1957–
When I'm gone : practical notes for those you leave behind / Kathleen Fraser.

Includes bibliographical references and index.
ISBN-13: 978-1-55046-514-3 (spiral)
ISBN-10: 1-55046-514-7 (spiral)

1. Family records. 2. Blank-books. I. Title.

CT9999.F72 2009   640   C2009-902042-4

Publisher Cataloging-in-Publication Data (U.S.)

Fraser, Kathleen, 1957–
When I'm gone : practical notes for those you leave behind / Kathleen Fraser.
[144] p. : ill.. ;   cm.
Includes bibliographical references and index.

Summary: A fill-in record book and resource manual to help family and friends better handle
the details of life when someone dies or has to be away from home for extended periods of time.
Includes space to give contact information, location of key documents, wills, living wills,
medical records, guardians for children, care of pets, finances and property,
home and vehicle maintenance, computer passwords, and special belongings.

ISBN-13: 978-1-55046-514-3 (spiral)
ISBN-10: 1-55046-514-7 (spiral)

1. Family records. I. Title.
640 dc22   CT9999.F737   2009

Digital linocut illustrations by Sue Todd. See www.suetodd.com.
Design by Gillian Stead

Printed in China

This book belongs to:

_____

_____

_____

Last updated:

_____

_____

_____

_____

_____

_____

_____

Contents

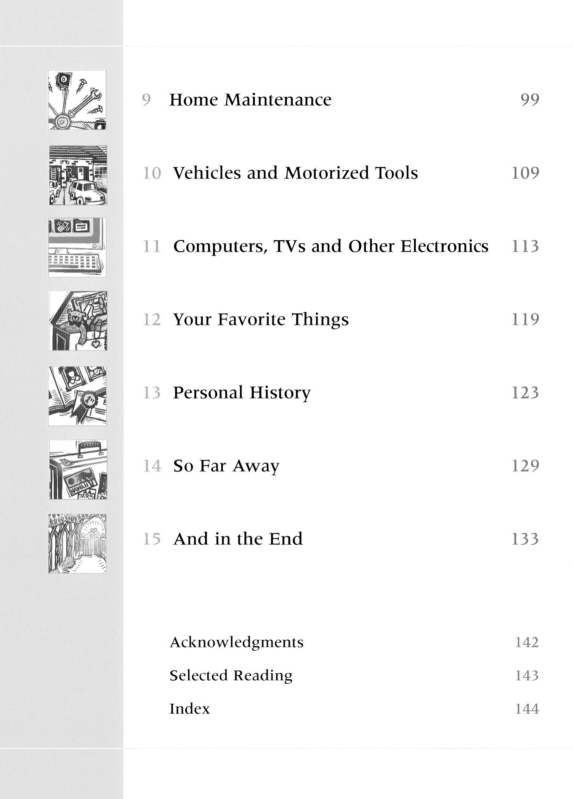

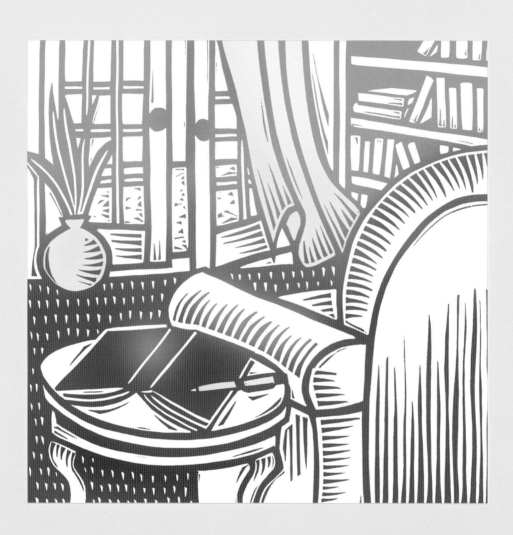

Introduction

Many of us have lost parents, partners or other family members and found ourselves suddenly without important banking information, house and car maintenance records, PIN numbers, the location of keys, codes, phone numbers, addresses and more. What if you were suddenly gone? If tomorrow you were run over by a bus, or diagnosed with terminal cancer or found yourself facing a debilitating illness such as Alzheimer's and you knew today that tomorrow you wouldn't be able to look after everything yourself any more? What if you are among the many people who, for one reason or another, have to be away from home for long periods of time — months, even years? How would your loved ones manage?

This is a fill-in book to give instructions to those who are left behind, not only on wills, funeral arrangements, insurance, lawyers and last wishes, but also on all the day-to-day details of your life and household and history, and what they'll need to know to carry on without you. It will be hard enough with you gone without their having to worry about who owes what to whom, what kind of medicine the dog needs, and how to clean out the pool filter. Almost everything they'll wish they could ask you when you are gone can be contained in these pages.

One of the basic ideas behind this book is you aren't going to live forever. Some day you are going to die. Wouldn't it be good to face that fact and be a little bit prepared? We prepare for all the other major events in our lives. Why not death?

Hand in hand with this idea is the notion that we really can't know what's around the corner. Even before you die, there may be a time, for one reason or another, that you won't be around to keep things running smoothly. You could be sick, you could be called up to serve your country in the military, or you could be sentenced to five years in the slammer for cooking the books. Or you may be suddenly divorced or separated, and sharing responsibility for children who will live away from you part of the time.

There will be things your family should know if anything happens to you — or to them. And there may be friends, neighbors and coworkers who depend on

WHEN I'M GONE — Practical Notes for Those You Leave Behind

you, and who will wish you had left them a few pointers on how to handle the day-to-day details. By ensuring all the practical information needed is available, and by making your wishes clear, you can better support others and provide for your own needs as well.

I have a friend whose husband is a long-distance truck driver. When their kids were young, her husband was on the road a lot and rarely home during the week. As it turned out, at the same time, her father, who had a farm in the country but a job in town, needed a home base in town for weekdays, and so he stayed with her during the week. For years! You can imagine, with three people running the household, that they had to devise a system for communicating everything to each other — what bills were paid, when the furnace filter needed replacing, when the kids had to register for clubs, and so on. If something had changed and any one of the three responsible adults in their home couldn't be there, a book like this would really come in handy. In other words, you don't have to be a morbid fatalist to use this book.

Although sooner or later, you will have to face death. As far as I can tell, apart from living a good life, there's not a lot you can do to plan for life after death. But knowing that your time in this life is limited, you can plan to make it easier for the people you care about to live without you when you're gone.

When my father died a few years ago, we were not at all prepared. It was a bit ironic that we were not ready, because his father and brother had both died at fifty of heart attacks, and so my parents considered every year Dad lived past his fiftieth birthday a bonus year. Mom and Dad resolved to do the things they wanted to do and spend time together enjoying each other. And they did — for more than twenty more years they were almost always in each other's company, leading a full and rich life. That year, as they did every year, my parents flew home to be with the family for Christmas. The next day Dad complained of a cold, so they went to the doctor, but the doctor didn't seem concerned. That night they went to a party with old friends and had a great time. But the next morning Dad was coughing blood. Mom called the ambulance, Dad was rushed to hospital, and by the end of the day he was dead.

We were all in shock. And since then, over past few years, we have had to adjust to Dad being gone. The biggest adjustment, of course, has been for my mother. She and Dad were less than a year away from their fiftieth wedding anniversary when he died. They had spent so much time together, grown up together, and depended on each other for so much. I don't know how Dad would have got along had Mom gone first — we joke that there would have been women waiting to snap him up and take care of him — but Mom was finding that the man she had married was irreplaceable.

Having just got through his funeral and a memorial, and all the myriad details of selling his company and winding up the estate, and having to do all the things my father had ordinarily taken care of for two households, and simply living through missing and mourning him, my mother was hit afresh by catastrophe. The summer after Dad died, their winter home in Florida was hit by a hurricane. The insurance company did not want to pay up and Mom had to deal with that and with tradesmen who seemed to treat her as an easy mark and would never, she was certain, have dealt with my father in the same way.

Dad kept extraordinarily complete and well-organized records about everything — in various files, or on his computer (although mostly accessible only through passwords or user names that Mom didn't know) — but there was still more that was in his head and never got written down, or if it did, we either couldn't find it or didn't know if what we found was the latest version. And without specific instructions, there was no way my mother was going to know how to operate all Dad's electronic and stereo equipment or, more important, if there were any other bank accounts or insurance policies she didn't know about. She certainly didn't have the receipt for the skylights at her fingertips when the first insurance adjustor tried to say the skylights were already leaking before the hurricane! She has come a long way since those early days, but there were many tears of frustration in the beginning.

My mother's frustration with all those everyday things after Dad was gone really affected her — and us. It made me and my husband think how disorganized we were, and how difficult it would be for our daughters to sort through our lives and belongings if we were gone. We had already been though the process and knew how stressful it was to deal with all kinds of unknowns when we were grieving.

We resolved to try to get ourselves organized. We're still only halfway there, but once I am finished writing this book, I promise to fill it in for our children, and to give a copy to my brother and sisters, and another to my mother, to encourage them to do the same. I may even give our daughters copies because, young as they are, they are beginning responsible lives of their own.

I do not mean to say that having a filled-in copy of this book will bring a loved one back home, or ease feelings of regret or grief. But I do hope that it will serve as a practical aid in what can be a time of emotional distress.

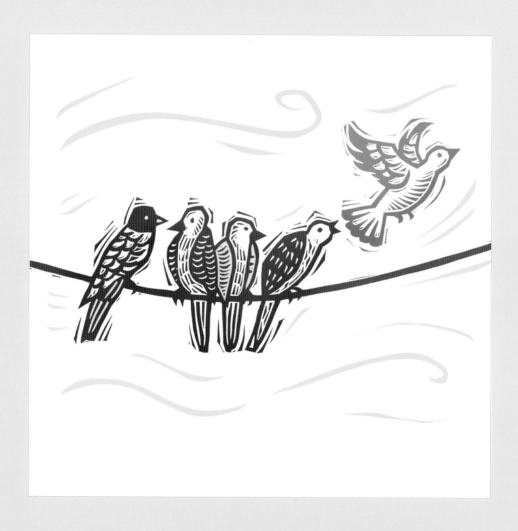

Important People

1

Perhaps you are a real social animal, the kind of person who has a large network of family and friends who keep track of and depend on each other. Or maybe you think of yourself as a loner or, more optimistically, a fabulously independent free spirit, tied down by no one, beholden to nobody. But think about it. Are there any people who count on you? Do you depend on anyone for anything? And remember, not all the people who are important to you are your best friends and mates. Once you start listing them, you might be surprised to find out just how many people there are in your life.

In this chapter you can provide contact information for all those important people, including the people who provide essential services to you and also those who depend on you. On the next page you will find a place to list those people who should be notified in an emergency.

Next of kin

In case of an emergency, when someone is injured or ill and needs to have someone notified, medical and other authorities will attempt to contact the next of kin. The next of kin may be needed to give information or consent in such an emergency. In the case of death, the next of kin is generally the person or people who must be notified and also take responsibility for the body of the person who has died. If you have no will or living will or power of attorney that names a responsible person, there has to be a way to decide who is your next of kin.

The definition of next of kin varies from place to place. Check with a qualified expert in your area to make sure you know who is or can legally be your next of kin and or represent you in matters of medical care or death. If you live abroad, be doubly careful to investigate this. The legal meaning of next of kin also has relevance if you die intestate (without a will) in determining who will inherit your estate. (See *Chapter 3, Legal Advice*.)

Emergency contacts

List emergency contacts in the order in which you would like them to be called and include information on how to reach them.

(1) _____

(2) _____

(3) _____

(4) _____

(5) _____

(6) _____

In the United States, next of kin refers to the nearest blood relatives of a person who has died, including any surviving spouse. If there is no will, it can mean any person who might inherit part of the estate by the laws of descent and distribution. Those laws vary from state to state on points such as whether or not stepchildren can be considered next of kin. In some jurisdictions, if you have no relatives, you can (while you are still living) nominate a close friend or other person to be your next of kin, and to speak on your behalf with doctors and others, and make arrangements for you after your death. Similarly, if you have died without relatives and without naming a next of kin, a close friend who has to register your death may be able to nominate themselves as next of kin.

The next of kin may be required to make decisions about your medical or other care if you are unable to do so in an emergency, and will have rights to make decisions about "the disposition of the body," but generally these decisions must be made in accordance with your stated or written wishes.

The Next of Kin Registry (NOKR) is a free emergency contact system operating in the United States and internationally to help if you or a family member is missing, injured or has died. It was developed by a man who, because of a nursing home's poor record-keeping, was not informed by staff of a nursing home that a family member had died. You can register yourself or family members with the NOKR through various law-enforcement agencies to make sure loved ones will be informed in case of injury, disappearance or death. Their website is www.nokr.org.

Although the fine print can vary from province to province, Canada is generally more liberal in recognizing untraditional unions, so you would think that common-law partners are more apt to have the same protection as legally married partners. However, that is not necessarily true. Nor is a stepchild automatically entitled to your property if you die without a will. If you want to leave property to a common-law partner or stepchildren, say so in your will.

In the United Kingdom, "Nearest Relative" is defined in the Mental Health Act 1983 to specify who is the person to be contacted and take responsibility for decisions as needed. This person is not chosen by the patient, but according to the order in which they appear on this list: husband or wife; son or daughter; father or mother; brother or sister; grandparent; grandchild; uncle or aunt; nephew or niece. Other people may qualify if a patient does not have a "nearest relative." The term Next of Kin is not defined by the National Health Service.

Who else needs to know?

I have friends from work and school and other realms of life that my family has never met. Even if my husband or children did know about them, they would have to work hard to track them down. And my mother has scores of friends that I hear about all the time — but I could not swear that I could reach them or even name them all.

Are there any particular people not included in your contacts list you would like to be notified in the event of your serious illness or death? Include their names and contact information and details about their connection to you:

13

WHEN I'M GONE — Practical Notes for Those You Leave Behind

Contact information

Include as much information as needed to make your listing useful, such as name, relationship, occupation, phone numbers, e-mail address, and home and or business address.

If you have relatives, friends and associates who change addresses, numbers, jobs and partners frequently, you'll want to review this information periodically, or at least make a note of where the most up-to-date information might be found.

Be sure to also note contact information for the people at your vacation or other home.

family doctor / physician

medical specialists

nursing service, therapists

hospital, medical clinic

other medical

dental

attorney / lawyer / legal advisor

> **NOTE:** Many of the people covered in this listing will feature in other parts of this book as well. For instance, your family doctor should also be listed with other medical professionals in the *Health and Medical Care* chapter. There will also be people not listed here who are covered in other chapters.

family _____

_____

_____

_____

_____

_____

ex-family (former spouse, in-laws, others) _____

_____

friends _____

_____

neighbors _____

_____

executor(s) _____

person(s) with power of attorney for health / for finances _____

guardian(s) for your minor children or other dependents _____

caseworker / contact for social assistance or other government programs

private health plan administrator _____

superintendent / property manager _____

employer _____

business associates _____

bank _____

_____

mortgage or loan holders _____

accountant / financial advisor / stockbroker _____

insurance rep / broker (life, health and home) _____

_____

babysitter / child care / parent / elder care _____

church / clergy / spiritual advisor _____

funeral home / association _____

taxi, bus or other transport service _____

Meals on Wheels or other home meal service _____

military association / veteran's administration _____

alumni association / sorority / fraternity _____

professional associations, organizations _____

social and recreational clubs _____

_____

volunteer organizations _____

health / fitness club / sports leagues, club _____

entertainment or sports team season's tickets _____

hair salon / barber / spa _____

therapist, physical trainer _____
veterinarian / pet sitter / kennel _____

pharmacy

grocery delivery

cleaning service

drycleaner, laundry service

magazine subscriptions

mail

newspaper delivery

library

lawn / yard maintenance

telephone service

computer / internet service

cable TV

water / sewer supply service

electrical supply service

heating / furnace / air-conditioning

security service

mechanic / garage / car dealership

painter, handyman, repair person

Memberships and affiliations

Where do you belong? Are there any membership accounts, fees, obligations or services that need to be attended to? Account names or passwords necessary to access information? Are you a leader or committee member? Provide contact information and other relevant details.

social, recreational _____

sporting, fitness _____

professional _____

corporate _____

union _____

education _____

religious _____

military _____

political _____

automobile associations _____

frequent flyer programs _____

library, book club _____

other clubs or associations _____

_____

_____

_____

_____

Do you have a gym or sports club locker? Where? What do you keep in it?
(See Keys and combinations on page 23.)

_____

_____

_____

_____

What if you have no family or friends?

For some reason there may be no one you want called if you get sick or die. You may have outlived everyone in your family, you may be an orphan in a new country, you may be estranged from your family, or you may just have lived a very solitary life. You may think you don't care, but not having any family or friends can complicate things when it comes to getting sick or dying.

Imagine a less-than-cheery scenario: suppose you fell ill or died and the only reason you were found is your landlord came to collect the rent. Depending on circumstances, events might proceed roughly in this order:

You're sick: the landlord calls emergency services and they pick you up and take you to hospital. You are treated until you are well enough to be released or until they find out you have no money or insurance. Hospital staff ask if you have anyone to take care of you at home. If you are lucky, they will find some charitable or other organization to help you out.

You're dead: the landlord calls emergency services or the police. Someone searches your things and questions your landlord and neighbors to see if they can find the names of anyone to call. They might look for an address book and check your mail and medicine cabinet. Police might contact the doctor who prescribed your medicine, but perhaps he knows nothing about you. You have no one to take over your assets and obligations, much less your body. Someone takes your body away to a willing funeral home or the city morgue. What happens then?

In Dickensian London, the bodies of orphans and paupers who died without family or friends with funds to bury them were buried "by the parish" in mass graves. In modern-day England, local councils still pick up the pieces of lives lived and ended alone: "According to Brenda Dickens, who oversees 300 public health funerals a year for Birmingham City Council, there is no such thing as a 'typical case.' One council reported burying someone who turned out to be a multi-millionaire." (Dan Bell, "All the Lonely People," *BBC News Magazine.)*

In Polk County, Florida, the Department of Health and Social Services arranges funerals for people without resources or relatives able to pay for them. There is no statutory deadline for waiting to find a next of kin, but the local health and social services manager says "...she doesn't recall ever having directed a body to be buried or cremated only to learn later of a living family member." ("The $575 Farewell," Gary White, *The Ledger.)*

If you are alone, take responsibility for yourself, make your notes and plans in a book such as this one, and then let someone know that your notes exist and where they can be found.

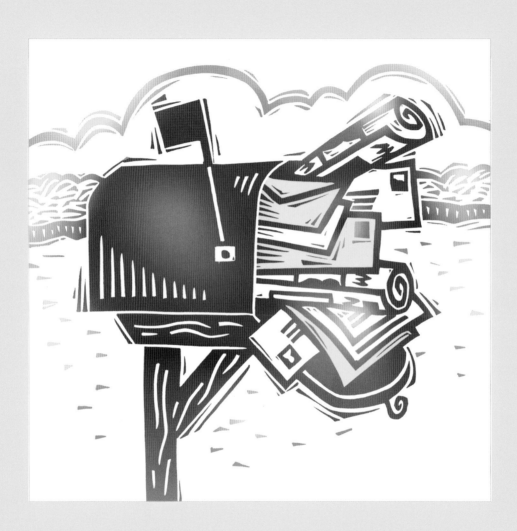

Documents and Records

2

Where do you keep important documents and records? Some people are meticulous record-keepers, and their important papers are all gathered together in clearly marked files in accordion folders, a new folder for each year. Others have no concept of how to file so they keep everything: papers stashed in boxes, files and drawers throughout their homes. And some people keep nothing — or they keep everything on their computers. If you were asked today to find your will, life insurance policy, cell phone contract and cable TV bill, where would you look? If someone else had to look for you, would they know where to start?

There are some documents that might seem unimportant now, but in a time of crisis can be critical. For instance, when a friend of mine died, his wife could not find their marriage certificate, and she had a great deal of trouble claiming pension and other benefits. Happily married for more than fifty years, I'm pretty sure they thought they were beyond the stage where they had to prove they were married!

In this chapter you can record the location of your important documents and records, and note any key information related to those documents. Getting your documents and records organized will not only help the people who may have to look after after your affairs when you are gone. It can be a huge weight off your own mind to know that you can find what you are looking for without having to turn your home upside down.

Use the next few pages to record the location of your important documents and records, plus any other relevant information. For instance, for your passport, you may note where it is to be found (safe deposit box) and also note your citizenship, passport number, full name, place and date of issue and expiry date. For your personal phone and address book, you might note "see this book / address book in kitchen in drawer under phone / computer e-mail contacts list." Be specific. None of this information is of any use to anyone if they can't find it.

Even if you don't have the actual documents, provide all the details you can. If you do have the originals (or copies), you can make a copy to tuck into the pocket at the back of this book and keep the originals in a safe deposit box or with your lawyer or in some other place known to the people who will need them.

Your documents and records

Many of the records and documents listed here are explored in further detail in other chapters. See especially *Legal Advice, Health and Medical Care,* and *Children and Other Dependents.*

passport / citizenship record

birth certificate

baptismal or other religious record

marriage certificate

divorce / separation papers

adoption records

custody / parenting agreements

your will

living will

organ donation card

power of attorney

banking, credit and other financial statements, cards, checks, receipts, bills health insurance information and cards _____

_____

_____

health records, yours and those of family members _____

_____

_____

government pension, benefits _____

_____

private/corporate pension, retirement, benefits _____

_____

life insurance, death or survivor benefits _____

_____

_____

Keys and combinations

The other day my young nephew asked me what all the keys on my key ring were for. Hmmm. There were the keys to my car, my husband's car, my daughter's car, to the front door of our house, to the back door, my locker at the club — and one to the old door we had before we replaced it, and one for my bike lock, and two for the office I used to work at but never go to any more, and one for the roof rack and…. Well, there were a couple I didn't have a clue what they were for. And then in the kitchen drawer there was another ring of different keys.

It is always a good idea to have one master set of keys clearly labeled and put away safely where they can be found if needed.

My master set of keys is located:

The key to my safe deposit box is located:

(For more about safe deposit boxes, see page 87).

If you have any combination lock — for example, on your bike, at the gym or on a storage locker — you can record the location and combination here.

My combination(s):

Do you have an in-home safe?

How to find lost bank accounts, insurance policies and more

Don't trust just anybody who says they'll help you find long-lost bank accounts for yourself or your spouse or other family member. There may be some legitimate businesses but there are plenty of scams out there, and if you are considering using a service, make sure the one you use is recommended by a reputable source. But if you have the time and energy, you may just want to do it yourself.

Banks, credit unions and insurance companies will usually make a good effort to help you find your own or your dear departed's accounts if you have a reasonable basis to believe that an account or policy does exist. Usually a person will bank in his or her own neighborhood or near a place of employment, so you can begin by searching the familiar and making inquiries there. Many people are creatures of habit and take their business to only one bank, although perhaps in different branches. You can also do a little detective work on your own — checking existing bank statements and or checkbook stubs to look for regular automatic withdrawals, for instance, to pay insurance premiums. Call credit card companies you regularly do business with to see if insurance policies were bought through them. If you do find a life insurance policy, ask to see the application form: it may include information about any other existing life insurance policies.

In the United States, the National Association of Unclaimed Property Administrators is worth looking into: they run a free website that gathers information from a variety of public sources and can give you further clues as to where to look for any money you may have not claimed. Check out www.missingmoney.com. They also have a good Links page that recommends other websites that may lead you to your unclaimed property, including dormant Swiss bank accounts, the IRS and the Department of Veterans Affairs.

In Canada, go to the Unclaimed Balances Service of the Bank of Canada to find your long-forgotten bank accounts, GIC deposits, term deposits and more. The Bank gets accounts only after there have been no deposits or withdrawals for at least ten years. Search online at their website: www.bank-banque-canada.ca/en/ucb/index.html. You can also contact the Government of Canada for assistance in tracing your own lost government savings bonds and certificates and, in some cases, transferring or redeeming certificates and or bonds of a person who has died to their beneficiaries.

In the United Kingdom, the British Bankers' Association (BBA) can help you find your lost bank, building society or NS&I account. Their free service is covered by *The Banking Code* and applies to every bank in the UK. Fill out an application form at www.mylostaccount.org.uk.

NOTE: *If for security sake you don't want to record certain information here, then at least record it where a responsible party can acquire that information — for example, with your lawyer, in your safe deposit box, with a security company, or with your sister.*

personal phone and address book and or contacts list _____

tax accounts, tax returns and records _____
_____

investment statements, other financial records / statements _____
_____
_____

property deeds, titles, surveys, building plans _____
_____

mortgage, rental, lease, condominium, cooperative housing or time-share
agreements _____
_____

credit cards _____
_____
_____
_____

other loan agreements, records of other obligations, current or discharged
_____
_____

home and other property insurance _____

employment records, contracts _____

self-employment and business records _____
_____

military service records, discharge, veteran's pension _____
_____

other government records _____
_____

driver's license / vehicle ownership / title papers / vehicle insurance policies

gun permits

instruction / maintenance manuals

account numbers, personal identification numbers (PINs) or passwords;
for example, for security systems or phone message or computer access
(See also *Chapter 11, Computers, TVs and Other Technology.*)

family records / family photographs

appraisals of any valuables, any list promising particular bequests to individuals

any other important documents and records

If there are any significant events or agreements for which you do not have records
or documents — for instance, if you have minor children but do not have copies of
their birth certificates — and you can acquire copies of them now, you should consider doing that. It will make life easier for you and for anyone who might have to look
after you or your obligations.

Keep or trash?

According to most professional organizers, all that paperwork can be divided into categories: (a) toss after one month; (b) toss after one calendar year; (c) keep for seven to ten years; and (d) keep indefinitely (forever).

Most pesky little bits of paper such as cash purchase and credit card receipts need to be kept only until you have recorded them or reconciled them with month-end statements, unless they are for a major purchase with a warranty or for a gift or other purchase that might have to be returned. If you run a home business, you may have to be more careful: anything related to business-use-of-home or employment expenses should be recorded and filed away. Monthly statements for bank, investment, credit and mortgage accounts and telephone and other utilities should be kept for a year — at least until after the annual statements arrive. Annual statements for these accounts and also income statements and forms and receipts for donations, education, medical expense, alimony, property taxes, etc., should be kept for up to ten years.

Tax agencies in North America advise taxpayers to keep tax returns, notices of assessment and any supporting documentation for at least six years. Business income tax returns, especially if you are self-employed, should be kept for as long as you are in business. In the United Kingdom, HM Revenue & Customs advises that you keep records of your tax and income for at least 22 months from the end of the tax year. Be sure to check what is required in your own corner of the world before you toss your tax records.

In your Keep Indefinitely/Forever file: birth, death, adoption, marriage and divorce certificates; child custody orders; education records; immunization and other important medical records; vehicle ownership and registration; original insurance and investment records; pension plan and military records; deeds to property; receipts for major purchases including appliances; will and power of attorney. There may, of course, be other documents and records vital to you and not mentioned here: use your own good judgment in deciding what to keep and what to get rid of.

When the time does come to trash your financial and other records, really trash them, even shred them. Whatever you do, don't put them out with the recycling! You don't want all your account numbers and private information strewn all over the street when a big wind comes.

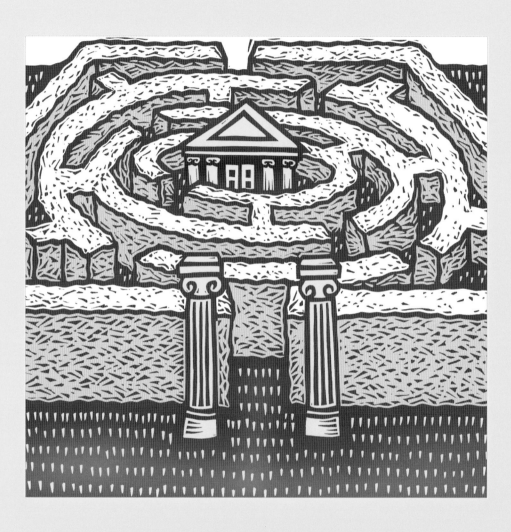

Legal Advice

3

The most useful and important bit of advice you'll find in this chapter — in this book — is this: write a will. No matter how large or small your fortune or family, you need a will. The pitfalls of dying without a will have already been touched on and will be further explored in this chapter.

The second-most important advice? Get proper legal counsel. Consult a lawyer or other legal expert when you are writing your will, power of attorney, advance medical directives and any other estate-planning documents. A lawyer can, among other things, help you avoid family squabbles. And minimize taxes. Consult a lawyer when entering into any major legal agreements, such as the purchase of a house or accepting a settlement for job dismissal. Yes, there are do-it-yourself kits for almost any legal situation, but they cannot give you all the information or advice that might cover your individual circumstances — and every situation is different. The law is a complex being that varies hugely in details and practice from place to place. However, do not allow yourself to be intimidated by the law or lawyers: like good manners, they have a purpose and can serve you well.

Described in this chapter are many of the legal documents you and your family may encounter or find a need for, especially in planning for your care should you be unable to take care of yourself. Some of the issues you should consider and questions you should ask yourself and others are raised. Use this chapter to record information about your will, other estate-planning documents, and any other past or existing legal agreements and obligations you have entered into. You can also use this space to make clear to your family your wishes and intentions in entering into particular legal agreements.

A brief legal history of you

Do you have a lawyer? Provide names and contact information for any lawyers you have worked with or recommend:

_____

_____

_____

_____

Are there any law firms or legal advisors you have used in the past that you wish to recommend _against_?

_____

_____

_____

How many legal agreements did you enter into today? Did you use your credit card? Your cell phone? Browse the internet? Borrow a book from the library? Those are just some of the ways in which you oblige yourself every day.

Some legal agreements, such as wills or property purchases, come to mind first. Others are not as obvious but can be equally important. Some agreements might never take the form of a written contract — for instance, if you are a freelancer, you may simply bill for time spent on each job — but you should still make note of them. Under _existing legal contracts,_ you might include any agreements you might have to supply or purchase goods or services, or contract or freelance employment, or long-term obligations.

Any legal agreements you have entered into that are worthy of note should be documented here. Include essential information, and provide greater details for any legal agreements not covered elsewhere in this book. Your who, what, when, where and why should include:

- the parties involved
- the date and place of the agreement
- the purpose and extent of any obligation
- any witnesses (if required)
- where related documents can be found
- any other details you think might be relevant.

Following this list and in later chapters are pages where you can make more extensive notes on your will, powers of attorney, living will and other important estate tools and documents.

your will (see also page 35) _____

_____

living will or other advance medical directive (see also *Chapter 4, Health and Medical Care*) _____

_____

power(s) of attorney (see also page 39 and *Chapter 7, Finances, and Chapter 4, Health and Medical Care)* _____

_____

trust(s) _____

_____

other estate documents _____

_____

adoption papers _____

_____

marriage, common-law marriage _____

_____

divorce _____

custody agreements _____

existing executorships (for instance, if you are executor for your sister) or power of attorney _____

_____

lawsuits, legal settlements and awards, past or ongoing _____

_____

worker's compensation _____

union or other labor organization agreements _____

employment contracts _____
copyright, royalties, trademarks or other intellectual property rights

ongoing court cases _____

military / veteran's service: history, obligations, rights, pension and other _____

criminal or other charges, history, sentences served or ongoing _____

outstanding fines, tax penalties, etc. _____

property titles (including joint ownership) (see also *Chapter 8, Property*) _____

cemetery plot, prearranged funeral services _____

property or other disputes or claims, lawsuits _____

debt-payment, promissory or other payment agreements not covered in
Chapter 7, Finances _____

service contracts (for home service, cell phone, other) _____

loans, including mortgages, given to family members or others _____

licenses for business, other operations _____

rental agreements or other property contracts _____

partnership agreements _____

business contracts _____

directorship _____

distribution rights _____

other business obligations _____

planned giving agreements _____

other existing legal contracts _____

Note that some of these agreements might be best detailed in the Property, Finances, *or other chapters of this book (see the table of contents). You can decide where is most appropriate.*

Do you have a family business?

There may be some aspects of your family-owned business that are relevant both to your personal life and legal affairs. Provide any important details here and also indicate where other information and records might be found if needed.

_____
_____
_____
_____

What happens if you die intestate?

Intestate means without a will. If you die without a will, you are going to leave your loved ones a lot of legal and financial wrangling as well as emotional turmoil. You have not appointed anyone to legally deal with your estate upon your death, so the court must step in and appoint an administrator or the public trustee. Your next of kin must apply to the court for the power to administer your estate. The court-appointed administrator must distribute your assets and pay your debts and taxes. If, for instance, there is no other surviving parent (if you and your spouse die together in an accident, for example), and no one else applies for the job, the public trustee becomes guardian and manager of the assets of your estate for your minor children, and government welfare services become guardian of your minor children for their care, health, education and upbringing. If you have no children or surviving spouse, everything might go to a long-lost relative you never liked...or to the government and the lawyers.

ORDER OF PRECEDENCE FOR INHERITANCE

In the absence of a spouse, a will or other clear directions, the generally — but not universally — accepted order of precedence is this:

- Children
- Parents
- Grandchildren
- Siblings
- Grandparent
- Great grandchild
- Niece / nephew
- Aunt / uncle
- Great grandparent
- Great niece / great nephew
- First cousin
- Great aunt / great uncle
- Great-great grandchild
- Great-great grandparent
- Great-grandnephews / nieces
- First cousins once removed (the children of first cousins and descendants of grandparents)
- First cousins once removed (the descendants of great grandparents)
- Great-grand uncles / aunts
- Great-great-great grandchild
- Great-great-great grandparent
- First cousin twice removed (the descendants of grandparents)
- Second cousin
- First cousin twice removed (the descendants of great-great grandparents)

Free legal advice?

Law societies and bar associations can advise you on where to look for low-cost or free legal assistance. For example, the Legal Aid Society in New York City works helps low-income New Yorkers by "resolving a full range of legal problems." Illinois Legal Aid (supported by the state bar association) has a guide to help you create a Power of Attorney for Health Care. In England and Wales, the Legal Services Commission runs a legal aid scheme to help people with civic legal problems or facing criminal charges. (See www.legalservices.gov.uk/.) Unfortunately, in many jurisdictions, legal aid cannot help you write your will. However, some other organizations, including law schools, will: for instance, the University of British Columbia Law Students Legal Advice Program will help people who qualify financially to write their wills.

Where is your will?

Make sure there is more than one copy of your will. Lawyers retire, people move and lose documents or forget where they have them filed. It's a good idea to ensure your executor(s), your lawyer and you each have a copy of your will. If you have a safe deposit box, put a copy of your will in it too.

Your will

Whatever you write in this book is NOT a substitute for a legal will. No matter how much or how little you possess, you should have an estate plan — and that includes a legal will. Many people just don't like to think about dying and don't want to plan for it. However, if you find yourself suddenly diagnosed with a terminal illness, you will wish you had planned ahead so you and your partner don't have to spend your final days talking to lawyers and worrying about the fine print.

If you already have a will, congratulations! Fill in the following information as best you can with as many details as will make it useful.

Who has copies of your will? _____

_____

Where are they? _____

_____

What form does your will take? _____
Executor(s) _____

_____

Lawyer _____
Date of creation _____
Date last updated _____
Additional notes _____

_____

_____

Special bequests

Whatever bequests appear in your legal will generally override any other written or oral promises you may have made. If there are heirlooms you want to distribute that *are not* specified in your will, you can list them by description, value and intended recipient in *Chapter 12, Your Favorite Things*.

If you wish, you can also use this space to list special bequests that *are* specified in your will (include name and contact information):

_____

_____

_____

Can I change my mind about bequests?

Yes, you can cancel your will and write a new one, or you can alter your existing will by making an amendment in a separate document, known as a codicil.

What does a will contain?

A typical simple will is generally organized like this:

Initial matters:

revokes former wills and codicils; appoints executors and trustees (often spouse) plus alternate(s) if spouse cannot do the job; okays fees for executor/trustee; survivorship; directions for disposition of body

Disposition of estate:

payment of debts; residue to spouse; alternate distribution (if no surviving spouse) to children in trust; to grandchildren in trust (if, for example, child is no longer living); if no spouse, children or grandchildren survive, to (for example) another person or people or charitable institution

Power to administer estate (gives trustees power):

to exercise property rights (deal with tenants, lawsuits, etc.); to realize and sell estate assets (converting assets into cash); to make payments to a minor beneficiary; to distribute in kind, that is, transfer assets to beneficiaries without converting them into cash; to invest the assets of the estate; to take steps to minimize taxes resulting from death; to employ others to carry out administration of estate and trusts; to decide if money earned or received by the estate is income or capital (important for tax considerations); to spend money from the estate for the maintenance, education, advancement or benefit of a beneficiary of the trust (for instance, for minor children not covered elsewhere); to retain services of a competent mediator or arbitrator if disputes break out; to borrow money for the estate; to manage, sell or lease any property and spend money as necessary to maintain and repair it; to represent estate as a shareholder; to carry on business; to incorporate a company to carry on business or hold assets of the estate

Guardianship of children:

appoint guardian (and name alternate); give trustees discretion to provide financial assistance to guardian to pay for housing and household help to feed, clothe, raise and educate minor children.

> Signature of willmaker
> Signatures of two witnesses

NOTE: For a will to be valid it must be signed, dated, witnessed by at least two people, and notarized.

About wills

The writing of a will is an art best handled by the experts. However, you are the person best qualified to describe your own circumstances and state what your wishes and intentions are in writing a will. What follows is a brief overview of some of the things you should know about when you are writing your will. This knowledge is, of course, also useful if you have to deal with someone else's will, as an executor of a new estate, for instance.

The executor

You must choose an executor to carry out your wishes as expressed in your will. Choose an individual you know and trust (family, friend), or a professional (lawyer, accountant), or a trust company (corporate executor) or, perhaps as an alternate, the public trustee. The executor must find all your assets, pay all your debts including taxes, and distribute assets to your beneficiaries either as a gift or in trust.

   You can name a sole executor or joint executors. If, for instance, you want your daughter to have the advice and assistance of your lawyer or accountant, you can make them joint, or co-executors. You should also name an alternate executor in case your first choice is unable or unwilling to do the job.

The executor's job is a big one. Responsibilities often include:

- Notification of death (to necessary people and institutions)
- Funeral arrangements
- Finding latest will
- Finding and inventorying all assets
- Determining value of assets at date of death
- Controlling, insuring and protecting assets
- Applying for insurance, pension, government and other benefits
- Preparing probate documents
- Opening an estate bank account, preparing estate accounts and having them approved by court if necessary
- Selling assets as needed
- Advertising for creditors and paying debts of estate
- Filing tax returns and paying taxes
- Locating beneficiaries and joint owners, and distributing assets as required
- Setting up and funding trusts as directed.

Note that your executor has no power to do anything until you die. If you want someone to make financial or health-care decisions for you while you are still living, you should prepare a durable power of attorney (see page 40) and a medical power of attorney, advance health-care directive or other similar document (see page 56 and also Chapter 4, Health and Medical Care).

If you choose to assign co-executors (joint executors), you should establish a way to for them to make decisions. For instance, if you choose your lawyer and your brother, or your son and daughter to be co-executors, do they each have an equal say in decisions? Is one person better qualified to make certain kinds of decisions? How should a decision be made if your co-executors do not agree? Are there certain conditions that must be satisfied? Might you choose one of your co-executors to have the final say? Or would you name a third person as arbiter? You should ask your lawyer to incorporate your thinking about your executors' decision-making in your will, but you can also record your expectations here:

_____

_____

_____

_____

_____

_____

_____

_____

_____

_____

_____

A second choice

Choose a second choice for beneficiary for your will, life insurance policy, and any other plan that provides benefits upon your death. Your second choice may become relevant in case of multiple death, if, for instance, you and your first choice of beneficiary die together in an accident. If there are no other particular people you wish to name, you can always choose a charity. In life insurance policies, you can designate "my estate" as your second choice for beneficiary.

The trustee

The executor and trustee are often one and the same person, but sometimes a will appoints a separate person or company to administer a trust for the beneficiaries of the will — for example, as trustee for your minor children.

If your assets are considerable and or have to be managed for a long time (for instance, if your child has disabilities or other challenges and is unlikely to be able to support himself even after he reaches the age of majority, or if your spouse is already in a nursing home and suffering from Alzheimer's), you may want to think about setting up an estate account with a trust company instead of appointing a member of your family to administer the trust.

The trustee's responsibilities include:

◆ investing the estate carefully and within limits of law

◆ following directions of the will

◆ keeping track of trust activities and balance, and being prepared to report on the trust

◆ making reasonable payments for care of dependents, as dictated by will

◆ making sure beneficiaries are treated fairly

◆ filing tax returns for trust

◆ knowing principles of trust law (to avoid conflicts of interest).

Consult your estate planning advisor about the different kinds of trusts that may be useful to you. For more about trusts and trust funds, see also *Chapter 7, Finances,* and *Chapter 5, Children and Other Dependents.*

Powers of Attorney

A power of attorney is a legal instrument devised to give another person authority to act as your legal representative and to make binding legal and financial decisions on your behalf. A power of attorney is usually prepared with a lawyer or other expert advisor, to designate your "attorney" — not meaning a lawyer, but a relative or friend or a trust company — to act as your agent and take over your affairs when you cannot.

Why do you need a power of attorney?

You may need a limited power of attorney if you are leaving the country for an extended period of time and want to give your spouse or some other person authority to sign documents on your behalf while you are away.

You will need a different type of power of attorney if you are unable to manage your own affairs because of illness, accident, disability or mental incapacity. It is a good idea to prepare both a medical and a general power of attorney. A medical power of attorney allows you to choose in advance a person to represent your interests and wishes and oversee your medical care when you cannot. A general power of attorney allows your loved ones to manage your financial affairs while you are unable to do so.

If you have *not* written up any powers of attorney, the court will appoint someone to look after your interests, medical and financial. The appointed representative(s) will be paid out of your estate and may not be a person you would have chosen.

Kinds of power of attorney

There are several kinds of power of attorney, known by different names in different places.

A **durable power of attorney** (also continuing or enduring) gives your designated agent authority to represent you until you die, even if you are physically or mentally incapable of managing your own affairs; however, you can revoke that power at any time. A **limited power of attorney** (also nondurable, or special) gives your agent power for a specified purpose or for a specific period of time, and is most often used outside of the country. It is useful when, for instance, you want someone to be able to sell property on your behalf when you are away. In most places, it is not valid if you become incapacitated. A **springing power of attorney** becomes effective at some future time, upon the occurrence of a specific event such as illness or disability.

Bank power of attorney can be required by your bank or financial institution; they usually have their own forms they want you to sign instead of simply accepting a power of attorney they didn't see signed and they also prefer not to accept limited powers of attorney, which expire after a particular date.

General power of attorney (or power of attorney for property) is usually created for the purpose of managing your assets and is almost always durable.

Your lawyer or other estate planning expert should be able to tell you which kind of powers of attorney are appropriate for you, for both financial and medical affairs, and especially taking into account their knowledge of the regulations and practices in your part of the world.

Medical power of attorney (or power of attorney for personal care) gives your agent authority to make decisions for your health or medical care in the event that you are unable to do so yourself because of physical or mental incapacity. A medical power of attorney is part of your advance medical directives, along with your living will. Note, however, that your attorney for medical care does not automatically have authority to override your wishes as expressed in your living will. See *Chapter 4, Health and Medical Care*, for more about how to use these tools to help your loved ones know what kinds of medical treatment you might choose or refuse if you could decide for yourself.

Choosing your "attorney"

Depending on the people available, you may choose a different person for your attorney for property and your attorney for medical care. The necessary skills and qualities may not all be combined in one person. For instance, your son may be experienced with finances and you may already rely on him for managing your assets, while your daughter may be closer to you personally, and a nurse, so more familiar with the medical system and your wishes and needs.

No matter what their particular responsibilities, your "attorneys" should be guided by the following principles. They should act honestly and in good faith for your benefit, mindful of your intentions and following the instructions you gave originally, unless it is impossible to do so. They should encourage you to participate in decisions to the best of your abilities, and choose the least restrictive or intrusive course of action when it comes to making changes. They should consult with other members of your family and friends who are sharing the work of caring for you. They should keep records of accounts and spending, and put your financial needs first, and next, those of your dependents, before other obligations.

As with choosing co-executors, if you choose more two or more people to be your "attorneys" you should specify who has power to make which decisions and also how decisions will be made if they cannot agree. The law almost always says that decisions must be made unanimously unless you have specified otherwise. Ideally, you will have chosen people who will be able to work together well and not end up struggling for control.

Your powers of attorney

Use the space on this page to describe in detail any powers of attorney you have created. Include this key information:

type of power of attorney _____

name and contact information of the lawyer or others who helped you create it

_____

_____

name and contact information of the agent(s) appointed _____

_____

_____

date of creation / date of revocation (if applicable) _____

where copies of the document can be found _____

_____

You can also describe the limits, responsibilities and authority given in it, but the best way for anyone to discover that information is to have the actual document in hand. If it is properly prepared with the assistance of a lawyer or other estate-planning professional, there will be no room for misinterpretation.

If you have created an advance medical directive such as a medical power of attorney, a power of attorney for personal care, a personal directive or a living will, you can record more about it in Chapter 4, Health and Medical Care, *at page 58.*

Death and taxes

As inevitable as death? Death taxes. One way or another, governments usually find a way to tax either the personal representatives of a person who has died or the beneficiaries of that person's estate. Consult with your estate or other financial planner to discover the best way to structure your estate to minimize estate and inheritance taxes, capital gains taxes, death duties and probate fees. Remember, however, that the first person to benefit from your retirement and estate planning should always be you!

What is probate? The meaning varies slightly from place to place, but generally, probate is the legal process of authenticating a will and distributing the estate. It proves that the will is valid and resolves claims and pays taxes. It confirms the executor's position as representative of the estate or, if there is no executor named, appoints one. For simpler estates, the probate process can take a few months — for more complicated estates, especially ones being contested, it can take years!

Can you avoid probate? Some property, such as life insurance, jointly owned property "with right of survivorship," joint tenancies, and property held in a "living trust" can avoid probate. There are ways to avoid probate by giving away property while you are alive, or by making more of your assets fit under the "probate-free" category. Consult an expert advisor.

Death and the law

When someone dies, the law sometimes pays attention in other ways besides estate law. See also *Chapter 15, And In the End,* for more about the procedures required by law after a death.

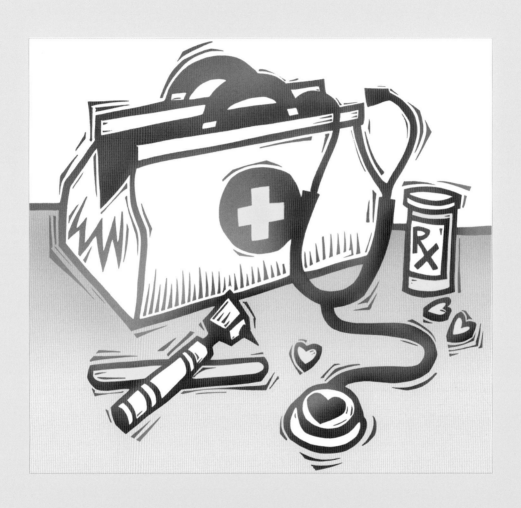

Health and Medical Care

4

I f we are lucky, when we are young, we hardly ever think about our health. As we get older, at least for some of us, there comes a certain fascination, perhaps even obsession, with staying healthy. This means more than learning new habits and breaking old ones. It can mean learning how to cope with or avoid doctors, medication, hospitals, surgery, medical bills and all that comes with a modern-day health-care system. No matter what your situation and your feelings about your health and the medical care you may or may not have received, you should have a complete health and medical record for yourself and anyone who may have to help take care of you.

In this chapter, there is space to record information about your health, health-care providers, health insurance, current health issues and a complete personal and family medical history. A family's health history can be a powerful predictor of possible future problems; sharing this information can help you ensure a longer, healthier future for yourself and your family. You can also provide details of any advance medical directives you may have created, such as a medical power of attorney and a living will.

Your health-care providers

Even the healthiest person will see many, many different health-care practitioners over the course of a lifetime. Fill in the space on the following pages with information about your health-care providers: begin with their names and contact information and the type of care they provide and where they provide it. If you can recall when you first saw them, and who referred you to them, record that information too. This listing can include everyone from your doctor to your pharmacist to the optician to the visiting nurse who checks in on you once every six months. You may have already included some of this information at the beginning of the book in *Chapter 1, Important People*. It's a good idea to repeat it here, and keep all your medical information handy in one chapter.

Your health-care providers

Name	Type of Care	Contact Information

POSSIBLE PROVIDERS:

family doctors (past and present)	gerontologist	physical trainer
clinic / hospital / emergency	gynecologist	physiotherapist
dentist	hearing-aid clinic	podiatrist
orthodontist	massage therapist	psychiatrist
allergist	naturalist / herbalist	other physical therapy
alternative health-care professional	neurologist	rheumatologist
cardiologist	obstetrician	surgeon
chiropractor	oncologist	other specialist
dentist	optometrist / optician	pharmacy
dermatologist	orthodontist	nursing or home-care services
ear, nose and throat	palliative care	respite care

contact person for health-care directives / living wills: (this could be the person who has your medical power of attorney, or your lawyer or the executor of your will, or some other appointed person.)

Location	Date First Seen	Referred by

Your health insurance providers

Most people get their health insurance from their employers or some other group to which they belong. All kinds of organizations, from alumni associations to automobile associations, offer members health insurance. That kind of insurance is almost always group insurance. An individual plan generally requires a physical examination, is more expensive and offers fewer benefits. Find out what kind of plan you have and what it covers before you end up in the emergency room!

Provide your:

policy or ID number, plan type and conditions, location of cards name of provider, employee benefits contact and contact information

names of family members or others who are covered under your plan

premium payments details

conditions

any other information you think might be relevant

Turn to *Chapter 7, Finances,* to record details about your life insurance.

Medical facilities

Provide information on the medical facilities you usually go to, including the closest emergency facility. Detail any emergency number and other contact names and numbers, plus location, with directions if necessary, and hours of operation.

Emergency

Hospital

Doctor's office

Walk-in clinic

After-hours clinic

Other medical facility

Pharmacy

(You can also include this information in *Chapter 1, Important People,* starting at page 16.)

Record of medical facility stays

Here you can record information on past or upcoming hospital or other medical facility stays. Provide the name of the facility, location, dates, length of stay, reasons for admittance, medications and or special treatment, doctor and other caregiver contact information, follow-up instructions and referrals. You can note the location of important documents and discharge papers or tuck them into the pocket at the back of this book.

- Hospital
- Rehabilitation clinic
- Mental care
- Nursing home
- Day-away or other adult recreation program

- Long-term care
- Convalescent care
- Hospice
- Group home
- Other

A brief health and medical history of you

In this space, record information about your health and medical history that will be useful to you and anyone wanting to help you if you are unable to do so. If describing an illness or medical problem, tell how long the problem has existed, any current treatments and any outcomes. Provide details as appropriate.

What is your blood type?

Was there anything unusual or difficult about your birth?

Have you ever had measles or mumps?

Have you had chicken pox or shingles?

Did you have any serious illnesses or injuries as a child?

Have you ever had high or low blood pressure?

Do you have a history of high cholesterol?

Do you have heart disease?

Do you have diabetes?

Have you ever had a stroke?

Have you had cancer?

Do you have any skin conditions that need attention?

Have you ever suffered from depression or other mental health problems?

Have you ever been pregnant?

Have you ever miscarried?

Have you given birth to any children?

Have you taken birth control or other hormone medications?

Have you ever broken any bones?

Do you have any tattoos, scars or other distinguishing marks on your body?

Are there any other ongoing conditions not yet described?

Describe any surgery: reason for, date of, place, doctor performing, result, etc.

Anesthetic history: Have you ever had a general anesthetic? Have you had any adverse reactions to an anesthetic?

Have you ever been in a serious accident and or suffered serious injury (broken bones, head injury, etc.)?

What inoculations/immunizations have you had?

Do you get the flu shot every year?
Have you ever been anywhere or had contact with anyone from whom you might have contracted an unusual disease?

When was your most recent tetanus shot?
Do you have an immunization record? Where is it?

Do you have an online personal health record? (see *Keeping Track* on page 54)

Where are your medical records kept?
Antibiotics: Have you ever had penicillin? Have you had any adverse reactions to any antibiotic?

Medical tests: Have you had any recent or significant medical tests (for example, X-rays, blood tests, MRIs, bone scans, etc.)? Detail the reason for tests, advising doctor, place, frequency, results and any other useful information.

_____

_____

_____

_____

_____

Medication: List past and current prescriptions, reason for use, prescribing doctor, dosage, first used, any ill effects. _____

_____

_____

_____

_____

_____

_____

_____

_____

_____

_____

_____

_____

Do you take any vitamins or herbal supplements? _____

Do you undergo or have you ever had any special medical or therapeutic treatments? _____

_____

_____

Do you have any allergies? What are they? Describe any adverse reactions.

Do you carry an EpiPen (epinephrine, also known as adrenaline) or other agent in case of allergic or other reaction?

Do you wear a MedicAlert or other bracelet or identifier? What is it for?

Are you a smoker?

Do you drink alcohol?

Do you take recreational drugs?

Do you or have you ever had any addiction to alcohol or drugs or other substance? Have you been treated for an addiction? What was the outcome?

Have you ever been given activity restrictions or told by your doctor not to participate in certain activities?

Do you have any genetic diseases? Have you undergone genetic testing?

Do you wear glasses and or contact lenses? Provide prescription information.

Do you have any medical or other implants?

Do you have a pacemaker?

Do you wear a hearing aid?

Do you use any other medical aids or assistive devices?

Have you ever suffered from gum disease?

Have you ever had teeth removed?

Do you have any special dental work (dentures, bridges, mouth guard, retainer, braces)?

Have you ever banked blood, sperm or tissue for possible future use?

Is there any other information about your health or medical history that might be of value?

Have you ever...?

Sometimes doctors have to be detectives. It can take seeing a pattern to help put two and two together. Check off any of the following symptoms that currently or regularly apply to you. If there is anything you check off here that you haven't already consulted a medical professional for, do so as soon as possible:

☐ headache	☐ blood in urine or bowel
☐ dizziness	☐ painful bowel movements
☐ sinus pain	☐ frequent urination
☐ earache	☐ frequent thirst
☐ difficulty hearing	☐ constipation
☐ fuzzy or blurred vision	☐ hair loss
☐ dry eyes	☐ leg cramps
☐ shortness of breath	☐ difficulty walking
☐ sore throat	☐ palpitations
☐ dry mouth	☐ numbness
☐ tooth pain	☐ tingling of extremities
☐ gum soreness	☐ unusual cold or hot feeling
☐ difficulty swallowing	☐ sudden weight loss or gain
☐ difficulty breathing	☐ depression
☐ stiff neck	☐ nervousness
☐ chest pain	☐ difficulty concentrating
☐ abdominal pain	

Keeping Track

It is a good idea to make sure someone knows what existing medical conditions or health problems you have and what medications you are taking or cannot take. For example, my immediate family knows that I am allergic to penicillin and have a heart murmur. A doctor should know that information in an emergency.

Recording the information in this book is a start, and that works well if you have contact information with you when you need assistance. Many pharmacies also offer a good record-keeping system and track drug allergies and even point out possible medication conflicts and contraindications. It is not always possible to go to the same pharmacy for all your prescription medicines, but it is best to do so whenever you can.

Some web-based services (such as www.ihealthrecord.com in the United States) and companies (Wal-Mart, for instance, for their employees) provide space to keep online personal health records. They can be accessed by those with passwords and also shared with health-care professionals. This can be particularly useful if you are sharing responsibility for someone else's care. If you use such a service keep a note about it handy, in this book and even in your wallet, so the information can be easily found when needed.

Family medical history

Is there any family history of health problems or medical issues that should be known by anyone taking care of you or your children or other dependents? Does your family have a history of heart disease or osteoporosis, for instance, or carry a greater risk for certain kinds of blood or other disorders?

Some family histories are more myth than fact. For instance, "My mother said her father was turned down by the army because he had a weak heart" may or may not be gospel, but often there is a grain of truth to the stories. Actual fact-based information about your family's health history could be very useful to family members and those who may assist in your care as well. Record any possibly relevant information here, noting who had it, their relationship to you and the details of the onset of the disease or condition.

> To record current health and medical information for any of your dependents, including children or elderly parents, as well as contact information for those who provide care for them, turn to *Chapter 5, Children and Other Dependents*.

Advance health-care directives

You can prepare legal documents to help ensure that your wishes will be respected if you are ill or in an accident and unable to speak or make reasoned decisions for yourself. These are advance health-care directives and usually consist of two different kinds of document, known by several different names but referred to here as a medical power of attorney and a living will.

A medical power of attorney (or durable power of attorney for health care, or designation of health-care surrogate, or health-care proxy) appoints someone you trust to be your representative in dealing with doctors and other care providers, to make sure you receive the kind of care you want, and to make medical decisions on your behalf the way you would want them made. You can specify what powers your representative has, but generally, your agent can consent to or refuse any medical treatment for you (with a few exceptions) as long as the decision does not run contrary to the wishes you expressed in your living will.

A living will (or declaration) tells doctors and other medical caregivers details about the kind of care you want to receive and do not want to receive if you become incapacitated. You can declare what steps, for instance, you want doctors to take to keep you alive if you are terminally ill, and when you would prefer to be taken off life support.

The subjects usually addressed in a living will are quality of life and end-of-life care. For instance, suppose you are close to death of a serious illness, in and out of consciousness, and a decision has to be made whether or not to perform surgery to prolong your life. You have stated in your living will that you do not want to have cardiopulmonary resuscitation (CPR) administered, or have to go through surgery, or be kept on dialysis or a respirator if those actions would prolong your life without any chance you would regain meaningful consciousness. You can specify which measures you want taken and which you do not.

You may also have declared that you do not want to have food and water artificially given when you are near death or unconscious. Permanently unconscious people can be kept alive for years with a feeding tube, but once that source is removed, they die quickly of dehydration. If you were to decide to refuse food and water you would be given medication to take away the pain.

No matter what you choose, an overriding assumption is that you want to be kept pain-free, unless you specifically state otherwise. Palliative care focuses on quality of life and keeping patients comfortable until life ends naturally.

Palliative care can be offered at home, in a hospice or at a hospital. Make your wishes known to your health-care providers and your agent for medical care.

See also *Chapter 15, And In the End,* starting at page 133, to make further notes on your last wishes when you know you are going to die.

When do your health-care directives take effect?

Your health-care directives take effect when your doctor judges that you are incapable of making your own health-care decisions. The determination of incapacity is usually made if you are unable to communicate your wishes or you cannot understand the choices available to you.

It is especially important to name a representative and to spell out what you want when you think family members might not understand or respect your wishes, or when you and your partner share a union not legally recognized as marriage. However, even in the most congenial families, there can be disputes among family members as to what constitutes appropriate care and what are extreme measures, so don't think that just because you and your family get along, they don't need you to put your wishes in writing.

Choose a representative you trust who will be able to stand up to for you to those who may not want to grant your wishes. Make sure that whoever you choose as your health-care agent either also has the right to manage your finances in case of your incapacity (i.e., has a durable power of attorney for property — see *Chapter 7, Legal Advice*), or else sees eye to eye with whomever you have chosen to give that responsibility. Name an alternate agent, in case your first choice is unable to fulfill the role. It is not usually a good idea to name your doctor or medical care provider as agent, as there can be a perception of conflict of interest.

If there is no one you trust to make medical decisions for you, you can still create an advance medical directive in the form of your living will. It will direct health-care professionals to follow your wishes and they may even appoint someone to care for you in the way you have requested. Just be sure to advise your doctor or other caregiver (for example, a representative at a hospital) that you have prepared a declaration of your wishes.

Most medical associations and hospitals and some doctors can advise you on what documents are accepted in your location and even provide forms for you to fill out for directing your own health care if you have not already done so with a lawyer. Health-care providers are required to respect your wishes and honor your representative's authority as long as the agent's directions are a reasonable interpretation of your wishes.

Make sure your documents are signed (or, if you are physically unable to sign them, have another person sign for you) in the presence of witnesses. Check with your local authorities to see what is required in your location to make your documents legal. There are also government and private registries that can make your medical directives available to those who might search for them. Ask your doctor if there are any suitable for you.

Your medical power of attorney

Do you have a medical power of attorney? _____

Who is your appointed agent? _____

_____

_____

When was it written and where? _____

_____

_____

What are the terms? _____

_____

_____

_____

Who witnessed it? _____

_____

Have you spoken to your doctor about it? _____

_____

Have you spoken to your family about it? _____

_____

Where is the original? Where are copies? _____

_____

Your living will

Do you have a living will? _____

When was it written and where? _____

_____

_____

Who witnessed it?

What are the terms?

Have you spoken to your doctor about it?

Have you spoken to your family about it?

Where is it? Where are copies?

DNR Order

A Do Not Resuscitate (DNR, or DNAR — Do Not Attempt Resuscitation) order tells emergency medical caregivers that you do not wish to receive life-prolonging treatment if your heart and breathing stop. This generally means that you do not want to receive CPR. (In some places it can also mean that intubation should not be attempted.)

You can make your DNR instructions part of your living will or a doctor or hospital representative should be able to help you prepare a DNR order. You can also obtain a MedicAlert bracelet or anklet to notify people that you have a DNR order. You can change your mind at any time about a DNR order!

Do you have a Do Not Resuscitate order? Is it part of you living will? Have you notified your doctor? Your family? Would you prefer NOT to have a DNR order?

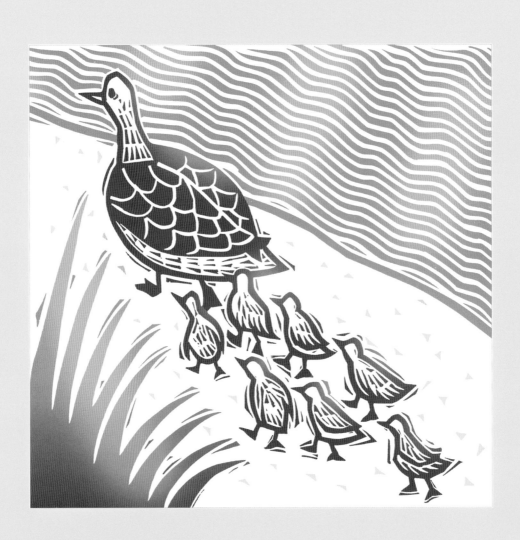

Children
and Other Dependents

5

A re there children in your life who depend on you? Do you provide care for any other people? Parents or other family members, friends or neighbors? Perhaps you feel responsible for them all. Undoubtedly you have thought about what would happen if you were no longer able or around to take care of them.

Your concern will be greatest for those people who cannot look after themselves, especially if you have responsibility for minor children. One of the hardest things to contemplate is leaving your children behind. You have likely already considered what might happen to your young children if you were to die or get sick or for some reason have to be separated from them. Perhaps you have an adult child who is facing difficult physical or mental challenges. Or you may have another kind of adult dependent, for instance, a spouse with dementia. A friend of mine has a middle-aged brother with Down syndrome who will need care and an advocate for the rest of his life. Who will look after them if you are not there? Who will know what is best for them? And how can you ensure that their property will be carefully managed and used wisely?

In this chapter, you can record information about all of those who benefit from your care.

The theme of the abandoned orphan has a great tradition in popular fiction. For many, the whole point of having a legal will is to make arrangements for their children in case an accident should happen and their children are suddenly orphaned. As parents, the two most important things you will do with your will are choose a personal guardian to raise your children and a property manager to take care of their property.

Choosing a personal guardian

When you are writing your will, one of the most difficult and essential decisions you will make is to choose legal guardians for your minor children and other dependents. Usually, when one parent dies, the other takes over custody and responsibility for the child. If both parents die, or a single parent dies, the court must appoint a personal guardian. In your will, you can name the person you would like to appoint as a personal guardian for your children or other dependents. The court always acts in the best interests of your child and will usually agree to your choice unless there is a good reason not to.

Obviously, if you and your partner are both making wills, you should each name the same person as guardian for your children. You should also have backup guardians for each child.

In choosing guardians, you will want to look for certain qualities. First, consider any family member or close friend of the family with whom your children already have a good relationship. You will find yourself balancing pros and cons. Your brother may be fine and upstanding but have three children of his own that he keeps on a tight leash. Your sister may be fun and easygoing, but on her third marriage and sixth apartment in six years. Your choice should be a mature and energetic adult who cares for your children and is willing and able to assume the responsibility of raising them in a safe and supportive home. You will likely want to cause the least amount of upheaval in your child's life. You may prefer to choose someone whose lifestyle, values, faith, and ideas about education coincide with yours. You'll also want to think about finances and living arrangements.

One thing you may want to stipulate is that whoever accepts guardianship of your children must take all of them and bring them up together. This can be a concern for large families with several children. Don't make assumptions. It may be that your children actually have stronger attachments to familiar adults than to each other. Perhaps your son is actually closer to Aunt Agnes than is your daughter, who may want to go live with her grandparents from your first marriage.

Talk to your prospects seriously about what they would be expected to do, judge their willingness to take on the role of guardian and, if your children are old enough, consider their wishes, and then decide. Your priority is to choose the guardian you think would be best able to care for each child.

When you are choosing a guardian for a dependent adult, you will have to find someone who is financially, mentally and physically able to take on that responsibility and also willing to do it. It can be a hard sell to convince anyone to take on an adult who needs round-the-clock care, especially if they don't already know and love that person. The brutal truth is, children tend to be more portable and malleable, and better suit the romantic stereotype of an orphan. Good luck!

Be sure to assign alternates and revisit assigning a guardian (and alternates) every few years as circumstances change.

Choosing a property manager

The role of a property manager is to manage the assets of an estate left to a child, including property inherited through a will, a living trust or life insurance policy, and property received from other sources. Children cannot legally own assets until they reach the age of majority. Any inheritance they receive must be held in trust until they are 18 (or 19, depending on where you live). The property manager has the authority to invest, hold or spend property in your child's best interest. Choose someone who is competent enough to deal with the property and who also understands your wishes for your children and shares or at least respects your values and ideas about how money should be spent.

When choosing a guardian for your minor children you will want someone you trust to raise them with your values and their best interests at heart. It is not unusual for the same person to take on the role of property manager, but your best choice for guardian is not necessarily the same person you might choose to look after your children's assets. In most places you can appoint different people for those different roles. If you do that, however, it is a good idea to choose people who will be able to get along, as they will be working in close collaboration to support your children in accordance with your wishes. It should be noted that you can name a guardian only in your will; you can name a property manager in your will, an insurance policy, a living trust or another trust.

In your will you can specify how you want your kids to inherit — a little at a time, or all at once — and that will help guide your agents in their decision-making. If, for instance, you decided you did not want your children to receive all of their inheritance at the sometimes reckless age of 18, you could set up a testamentary trust. Your property manager (the trustee of the trust) could then distribute funds to pay for their education and other expenses while they are minors, but not release any larger sums until they reached a certain age, or in installments, for instance, at age 21, 25 and 30. As with guardians, you should name an alternate property manager.

Dependent Children

In this first section, you can record information about your own minor children, adopted children, stepchildren, foster children, godchildren and any other young children for whom you regularly provide care, and any children for whom you have agreed to be guardian and or property manager in the event of their parents' death. Be sure to note the location and relevant details of any important documents, such as birth certificates, school, custody and medical records and your own estate documents. Fill in as much information as is relevant to you. *Make photocopies of these pages to record information for more children as needed. (A section follows for recording information about your independent adult children and any dependent adults.)*

Full name

Date and place of birth

Citizenship (also note location of birth certificate, passport, other citizenship papers)

Height, weight, eye color, hair color

Distinguishing marks (birthmarks, tattoos, scars)

Your relationship to child

Contact information for child

Residence

Other residence

Parents' names and date and place of birth

Adoption, foster care or other records

Custody, shared guardianship or co-parenting agreements

_____

_____

_____

Type of care you provide _____

_____

_____

_____

Other care provider or family member name(s) and contact information (include daycare, nursery school, babysitters) _____

_____

Personal guardian _____

Alternate guardian _____

Document in which guardian is named _____

Property manager _____

Alternate property manager _____

Document in which property manager is named _____

_____

_____

Health and medical information (see _Chapter 4, Heath and Medical Care,_ for the kind of information that may be relevant here)

Doctors' names and contact information _____

_____

_____

_____

Dentist, orthodontist _____

_____

Other medical professionals _____

_____

_____

Health insurance details

Blood type

Vaccinations and inoculations

Any childhood diseases, injuries

History of hospitalization, surgery

Ongoing conditions, treatment

Medical records, online personal health records

Medication (provide all necessary details)

Allergies

Glasses

Hearing aid, PM system for classroom use

Medical implants

Other assistive devices

Dental work, braces, retainer

Other

Diet preferences and requirements

Daily care and routines (weekdays, weekends, summers)

Schools, education history (include contact information, bus or other travel details, names of principals, favorite teachers and other key people, location of report cards and other records, awards, scholarships, important dates, tuition or other fees, etc.)

Responsibilities

Home safety precautions

Spiritual / religious development (faith and practice, customs, place of worship, contact information)

Recreation, sports, music, art, hobbies, lessons and other pastimes

Friends and social groups

Pets, pet care

Music, art, sports, hobbies, other interests

Other interests and accomplishments

Dependent Adults

Use these next few pages to record information about any adults who depend on you. For those whose lives and care truly depend on you, especially anyone for whom you have legal guardianship, you will want to fill in as much detailed information as you can.

As for your own grown and independent children, there are other places in this book where you can record your family history and family medical history, but some of the questions that appear here do not arise anywhere else, so you may choose to record their information here. (You may know things about your own grown children that even they don't know.)

> Make photocopies of these pages to record information for any other dependent or independent adults. There may also be some people for whom you do only small errands and chores, such as walking the dog or picking up the newspaper. Make notes on those people and errands in the "Small Favors" section immediately following this section at page 73.

Full name _____

Date and place of birth _____

Citizenship (also note location of birth certificate, passport, other citizenship papers) _____

Height, weight, eye color, hair color _____

Distinguishing marks (birthmarks, tattoos, scars) _____

Your relationship _____

Contact information _____

Residence _____

Other residence _____

Parents' names and date and place of birth

Spouse, partner and other family members (name, contact information)

Marriage, divorce, separation records

Adoption, foster care, custody, parenting or other records

If applicable:
Type of care you provide

Other care and service providers and contact information (include housekeeping, hairdressing, transportation and other services)

Personal guardian

Alternate guardian

Document in which guardian is named

Property manager
Alternate property manager
Document in which property manager is named

Health and medical information (see *Chapter 4, Heath and Medical Care,* for the kind of information that may be relevant here)

Doctors' names and contact information

_____

_____

Dentist / orthodontist _____

Other medical professionals and caregivers _____

_____

Health and disability insurance details _____

Medical records, online personal health records _____

Blood type _____

Vaccinations and inoculations _____

Any childhood diseases, injuries _____

History of hospitalization, surgery _____

_____

Ongoing conditions, treatment _____

Medication (provide all necessary details) _____

Glasses _____

Hearing aids _____

Medical implants _____

Other assistive devices _____

Dental work, dentures _____

_____

Allergies

Limits to activity, mobility

Mental limitations, competency

Addictions
Other

If applicable:
Diet preferences and requirements

Daily care and routines

Home safety precautions

Advocacy groups and community organizations

Pension, veteran's care and other benefit plans

Finances (income, investments, assets, liabilities, bank accounts, obligations, life and home insurance, including contact information)

Home and property

Education history, schools

Employment history, volunteer work and other responsibilities

Spiritual / religious needs (faith and practice, customs, place of worship, contact information) _____

_____

Friends and social groups _____

_____

_____

Music, art, sports, hobbies, other interests _____

_____

_____

Other interests and accomplishments _____

_____

See *Chapter 4, Health and Medical Records,* to read about online personal health records. These can be created for individual and families, added to or accessed by those with passwords, and also shared with doctors and other health-care professionals. You may want to consider creating an online profile if you are keeping track of dependents from afar or sharing that responsibility with siblings.

Do your dependents have wills of their own?

Even though an adult might be dependent on you for care, that does not mean that person does not need a will or advance medical directives.

Does your adult dependant have a legal will? Are you executor? If not, who is?
_____

Has your adult dependent written an advance medical directive (for instance, a medical power of attorney or living will)? _____

_____

Do you have power of attorney for your adult dependent?
_____

If not, who does? _____

If these documents exist, when were they prepared, by whom, and do you have copies? _____

Small Favors

This is where you can make notes on the people who depend on you for the little things, such as walking the dog, bringing lunch once a week, a trip to the grocery store or the library. Be sure to name any other care providers and contacts for the person you are assisting, in case you are ever unavailable and someone else has to fill in for you. And, yes, little things can mean a lot.

- Person's name, address and contact information
- Date of birth
- Your relationship
- Type of care you provide (include time and place and recurrence)
- Special interests, likes and dislikes
- Other care providers and contacts for the person

Caregivers

A caregiver is anyone who provides assistance to someone else who is in some way incapacitated and needs help. Family, friends and neighbors who are caregivers are rarely paid for the care they provide and may give hours of care while holding regular full- or part-time jobs.

You may not think of yourself as a caregiver, but do you ever do grocery runs for your aging parents? Do you regularly walk you neighbor's dog or drive your sister to the doctor? Perhaps you do take full-time care of an invalid or bring meals to a shut-in. You are not alone.

The numbers are staggering, and only increasing. In the United States, according to a 2003 Report to Congress quoted on the Family Caregiver Alliance website (www.caregiver.org), "Unpaid family caregivers will likely continue to be the largest source of long-term care services in the U.S. and are estimated to reach 37 million caregivers by 2050, an increase of 85% from 2000." Some organizations such as the Alzheimer's Association offer support groups for caregivers and offer a shared common experience. (The national Alzheimer's Association website offers a Caregiver's Stress Test: see www.alz.org/stresscheck/)

According to reports on the Victorian Order of Nurses Canada website (www.von.ca), the numbers in Canada are comparable (2.8 million caregivers in 2003), the stresses considerable, and the future will be even more challenging, especially given such factors as an aging population, fewer resources for paid care, and the "idealization of death at home and the pressure to provide care at home."

And according to the Carers UK website (ww.carersuk.org), one in eight adults (around 6 million people) in the United Kingdom are "carers," and they estimate that by 2037, the number will increase to 9 million. Among the goals of this organization are more public funds, more flexible work arrangements, and greater recognition for caregivers.

If you are taking care of someone, especially an adult dependent, and finding it too much to deal with, get help. You do not have to do it all on your own. Turn to your local government agencies, hospital, doctors, advocacy, community and church groups for help and advice. All of the websites mentioned above are good resources and provide links to other sources of information, advocacy groups and support for caregivers.

All my children

My daughters always enjoy hearing about themselves as babies — if they were good sleepers, if they cried a lot, who they looked like, what they liked. Imagine that you are the only person who remembers your children when they were young; they may long to know about moments you shared with them and memories only you can provide.

Use this space to tell stories about any children you care for and have responsibility for. These may be your own children or any other children whose lives are connected to yours. Some things you may want to write about will include:

- Favorite foods
- Favorite TV shows / movies / games / music / books / sports teams
- Likes and dislikes
- Fears
- Special interests
- Strengths
- Talents, skills
- Languages, musical abilities

- Weaknesses, conflicts, bad habits
- Friends (young and adult)
- Connection to you
- Holidays
- Travel, special outings
- Favorite possessions
- Ambitions, dreams
- Worst memories
- Favorite memories

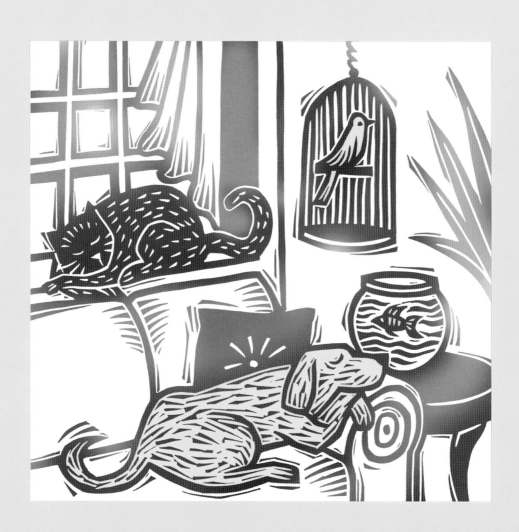

Pets

6

If you have ever had a pet, you will know that pets quickly become valued members of the family. Companions in good times and bad, pets offer us unconditional love and depend on us for everything. If you have a pet, you will want to know that if you are not there to provide care, your beloved animal will continue to receive the same loving attention that you have always provided.

Different choices will arise for different circumstances. You may have to make decisions about the care of a younger animal while you are away on long-term, long-distance work assignments. You may have to go into a care facility where pets are not allowed, and need to find a home and caregiver for an animal companion of many years. Or you may have just learned that you do not have long to live, and be unable to find anyone who is willing to take over the care of your beloved but aging pet.

This chapter provides a place to make known your wishes for your pet — or pets — and to provide information about the care of your companion animal. It also explores some of the resources and options open to you, including pet sitting, boarding, rescue centers, pet adoption, humane societies, pet cemeteries and more.

Pets are a long-term commitment. Dogs will live anywhere from about 8 years to almost 20 years, depending on size, breed and the lifestyle and care they enjoy. "Outdoor" cats have shorter lives than "indoor" cats: compare about 6 years to 16 years. Aquarium fish live 5 to 10 years, and some goldfish can keep on swimming up to 30 years. Budgies might live for 15 years. Parrots have been known to outlive their owners: a well-cared for African Grey can live for 50 years. Pet lizards can live for 10 to 20 years. A healthy horse has a life expectancy of 25 years or more.

You will want to make sure that your pets are provided the same care and attention you would give them if you could. Record important information about the animals you love here, so that anyone who has to take over for you will be well prepared.

Your Pets

◆ name(s)

◆ birth date(s) / age(s)

◆ breed(s), breeding history, breeder contact information

◆ license, registration, ID tattoo or other

◆ location of important documents

◆ vet's name and contact information

◆ food, treats, other requirements

◆ health history, medical records • vaccination, shots • medication, vitamins (schedule, names, dosage) • health concerns

◈ daily routine, exercise schedule • pet park or other recreation location • other pet friends • fears and habits _____

◈ pet sitter, day care • emergency care • boarding (kennel or other) • grooming services • aquarium service • special care, treatments

◈ gear (grooming, other) • favorite toys, bed, blanket, other • transport, cage, carrier, enclosure, electric fence _____

◈ Do you belong to any pet training, breeder associations or kennel clubs? Do you breed your animals? What honors has your pet won?

If you have more than one pet and a lot more information to record, make photocopies of these pages to include here.

Finding a pet sitter

Pet sitters are professionals paid to visit your home to look after and spend time with your pet. A good pet sitter makes sure food and water are available, gives your pet exercise, and knows how to tell if your pet needs the attention of a veterinarian. Some pet sitters also offer additional services, such as bringing in mail and newspapers, watering plants, turning lights on and off, and otherwise making your home looked lived in while you are away in order to deter crime. The benefits for your pet include a familiar, safe home, a regular diet and routine, individual attention, and no stress because of travel, change and other animals.

Begin your search for a pet sitter by seeking out recommendations from your vet, dog trainer, friends and neighbors. Ask if you can have a home interview with your pet present, so you can judge if the sitter seems confident and competent.

There are a few ways you can help prepare your pet and pet sitter for your absence:

◆ Do what you can to ensure your pet is well-socialized.
◆ Leave food, dish, medication, bed, cage, lead or whatever supplies are needed in agreed-upon places. Make sure you have enough food and medicine for as long as you plan to be away and longer.
◆ Make sure records and vaccinations are up to date and your pet has all current tags and identification.
◆ Leave written instructions and contact information for you and your vet.
◆ Give a trusted neighbor a key to your home and the name and number of your pet sitter, and give your sitter the neighbors's contact information, in case of unforeseen mishap.

Evaluating a pet care or boarding facility

Dog boarding kennels, catteries, other overnight boarding services and pet daycare centers are all options. Ask questions before you commit:

◆ Where will your pet stay and sleep? Ask to see the space and judge for yourself if it is clean and comfortable.
◆ Can you provide your own food? Will the facility provide food or treats? How is water made available?
◆ How and when is exercise provided? Will your pet get time outside? What about when it is raining, very hot or very cold?

- How much of the time will your pet be personally supervised? Can you arrange for individual play and grooming time?
- Is there a monitoring system? Are there safety barriers to prevent "escapes"?
- Can the facility ensure all animals boarded are free of communicable diseases?
- How will your pet be separated from other animals?
- Will the facility keep records on your pet's health and behavior? Will staff contact you if your pet becomes ill?

Pets in nursing homes and other care facilities

There has been quite a bit of publicity surrounding animal therapy at nursing homes and other care facilities. In particular, a press favorite is the story of the nursing home cat, "Oscar, the furry grim reaper," who would predict a patient's demise, doing his rounds but singling out particular patients and sitting with them a few hours before they died.

But the good news about animal therapy is the positive physiological, emotional and spiritual outcomes that result. Many hospitals and nursing homes have therapy animal visitation programs and others actually allow patients to be visited by their own pets. If you are in hospital for recovery or rehabilitation for a long time, a visit from your pet may be just the thing you need to lift your spirits and also reassure you that your pet is being well looked after.

Plans for your pet

Have you made any care plans for your pet(s)? _____

_____

_____

_____

If your pet needs medical treatment while you are away, what are your wishes?

_____

_____

_____

_____

_____

_____

Pet insurance

The cost of vet services can be considerable, even for a healthy animal. As your pet gets older, you may find there are increased medical costs. Pet insurance is an option for some people, but you should carefully study the fine print in any pet insurance policy before you sign on the dotted line. See also www.spca.com/pages/insurance for more information.

A few questions to ask and things to watch out for:

- What are the policy limits and deductible?
- What does the plan cover? Illness, accident, chronic diseases? Routine care and diagnostics? Teeth cleaning? Yearly visits? Surgery?
- What is the likelihood your pet will need special care?
- Can you use your own vet? Do they recommend the company and policy?
- Will emergency services elsewhere be covered?

Do you have pet insurance? Document any pet insurance policy, terms, claims or other information here:

Giving up your pet

In the event that you have been told or come to realize that you can no longer care for your pet, there are options. You can advertise among your friends and associates for a good home for your pet. Ask your vet or local humane society if they can help. There are rescue organizations (some breed specific, some not), pet shelters, national and local humane societies and more. There are also organizations such as Petfinder (see www.petfinder.com) "temporary home of 272,490 adoptable pets from 12,452 adoption groups." Through Petfinder, interested people can adopt a pet, search for adoptable pets, find adoption groups, and post a pet classified ad by breed.

Where do you want your pet(s) to go if you can no longer provide a home or care? Do you have a guardian in mind? Has that person agreed to care for your pet?

Have you set aside any funds for the purpose of paying for your pet's care?

Is there a special pet shelter, rescue organization or other other animal welfare group to which you wish to make a donation? Have you noted this information in your will?

At what point would you be prepared to have your pet "put down"? When your veterinarian recommends it? If you are no longer able to provide a home and care? Have you discussed your wishes with your vet, family and or friends? What plans have you made in advance, if any?

What if your pet dies?

If your pet dies while you are away or while in the care of someone else after your death, what are your wishes? Have you made any prearrangements? As with your own arrangements after death, there are many choices available and there is no right or wrong.

Check with your veterinarian or pet "aftercare" provider for advice. The International Association of Pet Cemeteries and Crematories (IAPCC) and the Association of Private Pet Cemeteries and Crematoria (UK) are good sources of information and provide links to their members: see www.iaopc.com and www.appcc.org.uk.

Can you be buried with your pet?

Most jurisdictions in the North America and the United Kingdom presently forbid the interring of animal remains in human cemeteries. That does not mean, however, that it doesn't happen. People have had the ashes of their beloved pet smuggled into the casket in the form of a small pillow or other receptacle. One funeral home owner suggested that although they are obliged to say no when asked permission to bury your aunt with her deceased cat, if your aunt has a favorite purse buried alongside her, no one on their staff would look inside it! Alternatively, there are some people who have legally had their ashes interred alongside their pets — in a pet cemetery.

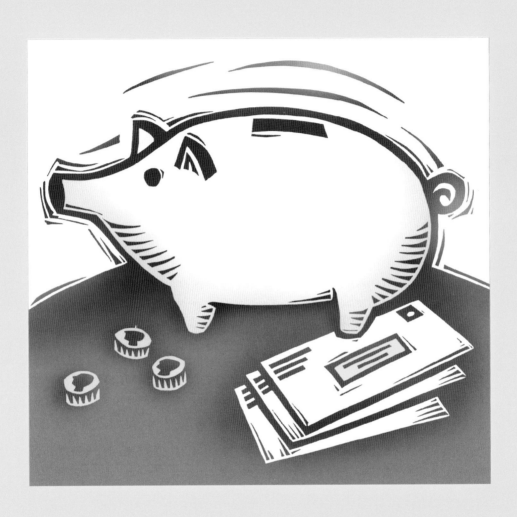

Finances

7

When it comes to financial planning, knowing what you have is essential. In giving you space to record your assets, liabilities, insurance coverage, taxes and other financial obligations, this chapter will help you to get the whole financial picture. The information you gather here will aid you in budgeting and planning ahead, keeping track of your progress and creating an estate plan. It will also be invaluable to anyone else who has to deal with your finances, including family and financial consultants.

Financial consultants

Provide details about any financial consultants you work with, including name, contact information, company name and the service they provide to you, plus notes on fees and statements.

_____

_____

_____

_____

_____

_____

_____

Assets and liabilities

Note all the details of your assets and liabilities on the following pages. If there is anyone with whom you share bank accounts, credit cards, loans or signing privileges, make note of that. Note where the paperwork can be found, who else has access to it, and if you have appointed power of attorney for any of the accounts or assets listed here.

Bank, other deposit accounts For each account include name of institution, branch location, account type, account number, web access information, PIN number or clue for internet or phone access, contact information. Indicate also if any of these are joint accounts and provide details. Note also the location of cards, checkbooks, passbooks, statements, checks ready to be cashed, and any other relevant items. Be sure to note any preauthorized payments and direct deposits for each account!

Employment income Provide details including employer or company names, employee number, contact information, account numbers, length of employment, location of relevant documents and information.

JOINT ACCOUNTS

Most people think they will have immediate unlimited access to a joint account if anything happens to a partner. But in some jurisdictions even a joint account can be frozen, denying access to funds by the survivor. Is your account joint with right of survivorship? Talk to your banker and or estate planner to determine what will best serve your circumstances.

SAFE DEPOSIT BOX

Do you have a safe deposit box? Where? What do you keep in it? Who has a key? Where is/are the key(s)? (See also *Keys and combinations* on page 23.)

_____

_____

_____

Note: As a general rule, do not keep anything in your safe deposit box that you will need in an emergency, particularly critical documents such as powers of attorney, your will or living will, or burial or funeral instructions, unless you have other copies elsewhere. This precaution is necessary because a safe deposit box is often sealed at the time of a person's death.

Self-employed, professional, contract and or other business income

Provide details including kind of business, company name, contact information for associates, account numbers, any other necessary information. Indicate where relevant documents and more complete information can be found.

_____

_____

_____

Investments List accounts that hold stocks, bonds, annuities, mutual funds and other investments. Include name of institution, location, investment type, account number, any regular payments or direct deposits, web access information, PIN number or clue for internet or phone access, contact information and location of relevant documents.

_____

_____

_____

_____

_____

Government assistance Provide details including kind of assistance, account numbers, contact information, account access, policy regarding renewals, application, etc. Note where any relevant cards or documents can be found. See also *Retirement, pension and savings plans,* below.

About government assistance

Government pensions vary from place to place, but there are similarities between most government-sponsored old age and social insurance programs. One common denominator is that the payments don't just start pouring in once you hit a magic age — you must apply for benefits. Do your research and find out what you are entitled to receive.

Retirement, pension and savings plans Include private or government pension, retirement, survivor benefit, investment or savings plans not covered elsewhere. Provide details.

Other income

Credit cards, store cards and other charge accounts For each account include name of institution, location, card/account type, card/account number, payment method, web access information, PIN number or clue for internet or phone access, contact information. Don't forget department store, service station and gasoline accounts. Note where cards and statements can be found.

E-bills, on-line accounts for goods or services, eBay and PayPal accounts Are there some accounts for which you have only online records? Record service or account type, account number, payment method, password, PIN number or clue for access, contact information and any other necessary details.

Charitable giving

Do you contribute regularly to any registered charities? Do you wish to continue those donations? Do you want any charitable donations to be made in your name in the event of your death?

Mortgages, loans, lines of credit For each loan or line of credit, include name of institution, location, loan type, account number, payment procedure and date, web access information, PIN number or password for internet or phone access, date of renewal or completion, contact information and location of documents. Be sure to note if any of these loans are insured.

Rentals, leases and other property payments and obligations Include rental payments, condominium fees, car loans, car lease, other equipment or property lease, other property payment. Note contacts and location of documents. See also *Chapter 8, Property*.

Other debts Include loans from family members and other personal loans.

What happens to my debts when I die?

Debts, including funeral expenses and taxes, are paid out of a person's estate. If the executor or personal representative does not know all of the people owed money by the person who has died, he or she must advertise for creditors to come forward and make a claim against the estate. These are the notices to creditors you see in the newspaper. If there isn't enough money to go round, your creditors may end up suing your estate for payment. Consult with your estate advisor.

> ## LOAN INSURANCE
>
> Remember that some institutions offer credit cards and loan agreements with health or life insurance to guarantee payment of the balance. (Some also offer insurance on your purchases, which is a different thing.) Check with your card or loan issuer to see what is covered and whether it is worth investing.
>
> If you are acting as an executor of an estate or as a caregiver for someone no longer able to take care of their own affairs, be sure to ask, when reviewing their credit cards and loans, if the cardholder or loan recipient had insurance to cover the balance owing in case of disability or death.

Insurance

"A man called on me the other day with the idea of insuring my life. Now, I detest life-insurance agents; they always argue that I shall some day die, which is not so. I have been insured a great many times, for about a month at a time, but have had no luck with it at all." —Stephen Leacock, "Insurance up to Date" in *Literary Lapses*, 1910.

You may be protected by various kinds of insurance through your employer or other organization, you may pay for your own individual insurance, or you may rely entirely on government protection and plans. Or you may depend on a combination of all three.

For each kind of insurance, note who and or what is covered, important terms, policy numbers and beneficiaries, how payments are made, contact information for broker and or agents, location of documents, benefit booklets and any other useful information. (See also *Chapter 4, Health and Medical Care, Chapter 8, Property,* and *Chapter 10, Vehicles and Motorized Tools*.) Remember to keep your information current — update it as it changes.

Life

Health / dental / disability

Travel, out-of-country

Property

Vehicle

Personal liability

Other insurance

Taxes

"What is the difference between a taxidermist and a tax collector? The taxidermist takes only your skin."— Mark Twain, *Notebook,* 1902

Property tax

Provide details about any property taxes or levies you pay. Include address, contact information, location of documents and receipts.

Personal income tax

If you are looking for past tax records and cannot find them, you can usually order them, for a fee, from the appropriate agency (Internal Revenue Service, www.irs.gov / Canada Revenue Agency, www.cra-arc.gc.ca / HM Revenue & Customs, www.hmrc.gov.uk).

How do you file your personal income tax return? By mail? On line?

Who usually prepares your return? Do you use an accountant or tax firm to help prepare your return?

Where do you keep your tax returns and other tax records?

Where do you generally have tax refunds sent? How do you generally pay tax owing? Do you pay in installments?

Are you entitled to a sales tax refund?
Do you also file a business or self-employed return?

Are you up-to-date in filing your personal income tax returns? Do you owe back taxes?

Have you ever been audited?

Other taxes (estate, sales, etc.)

Provide details about any other taxes, levies or government fees you pay or have paid, or tax or other government refunds you receive. Note location of relevant documents and receipts.

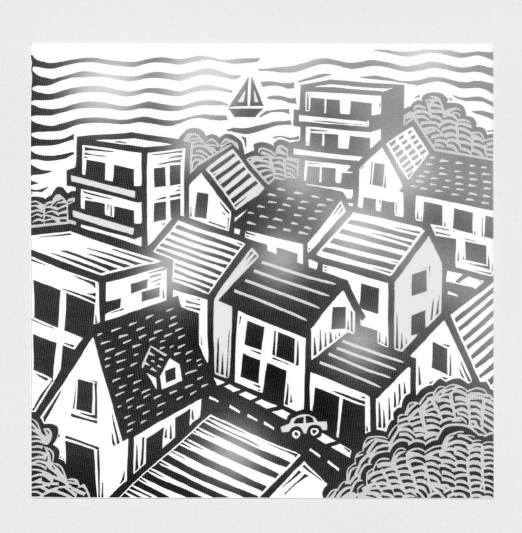

Property

8

To the average person, "my property" is the land that belongs to me — my house, my land, my real estate. Private Property: No Trespassing! And that is the broad meaning given to the word "property" in this chapter.

On the next few pages you will have space to list all the real estate that you own, rent, lease, share or otherwise have claim to or responsibilities for. You can also record information and your thoughts on your vacation property, should you be so lucky as to own a home away from home.

To record information about living in and maintaining your primary and any secondary home, turn to *Chapter 9, Home Maintenance.*

My property

Provide details, including address, ownership, location(s), buildings and other structures, date of purchase, price or cost, name of seller or lessor, terms of rental or lease, property tax information and any other relevant information.

What records do you have for these properties (deeds, rental or lease agreements, land surveys, mortgages, wills, contracts, etc.) and where are they kept?

_____

_____

_____

_____

What property obligations do you have, financial or otherwise?

_____

_____

_____

Do you have a share in any business or other financial venture? What is your share? What are your obligations? Who are your partners?

_____

_____

_____

_____

Do you own or rent a storage locker, garage or other place not already listed where belongings are stored? Where is it and how can it be accessed?

_____

_____

_____

_____

To record information about property insurance, see page 92 in _Chapter 7, Finances_.

Vacation property

Are you are lucky enough to have a vacation property — a home away from home where you can relax and enjoy a change from everyday life? Vacation property ownership can get complicated for various reasons, including death and taxes and family dynamics, especially when a property is shared. You will likely have your own ideas about how you want your vacation home to function, whom you want to share it with and what you want to happen to it when you are gone.

This is the place to record those thoughts, as well as basic information about your ownership or share of ownership of the property:

_____

_____

_____

_____

_____

_____

What will happen to your vacation home?

Vacation homes are more apt to be handed down through the family than primary residences. Speak frankly about your plans with all family members, individually and together, before you make your decisions about how to deal with a vacation property. Handing down of vacation homes is more complicated than ever because of practical, legal and financial difficulties, including taxes and rising real estate prices.

You may choose to sell your holiday home to your children now, if you can no longer afford to keep it or want the money to do other things. There may be circumstances in which you decide to "gift" your property to your offspring during your lifetime — for tax purposes, to transfer the burdens of ownership to them, including costs of operating, and to avoid probate. If you are gifting, you should make sure you can continue to have use of it, and keep it from being sold or mortgaged.

In some jurisdictions, *inter vivos* (living) trusts can be used, in which ownership of the property is transferred to a trust while parents are still alive, so capital gains tax is not payable until the property is conveyed to the heirs. Testamentary trusts can be created to leave funds to be used exclusively for the purposes of maintaining the property if, for instance, the heirs do not all have funds themselves to pay taxes and other large expenses such as replacing the roof. This is especially useful when a vacation home is left to descendents with varying incomes and financial circumstances.

Laws vary from place to place, so the advice of an estate planner and tax accountant are recommended. See also the bibliography at the end of this book for resources on this subject, including Douglas Hunter's *The Cottage Ownership Guide: How to Buy, Sell, Rent, Share, Hand Down & Retire to Your Waterfront Getaway.*

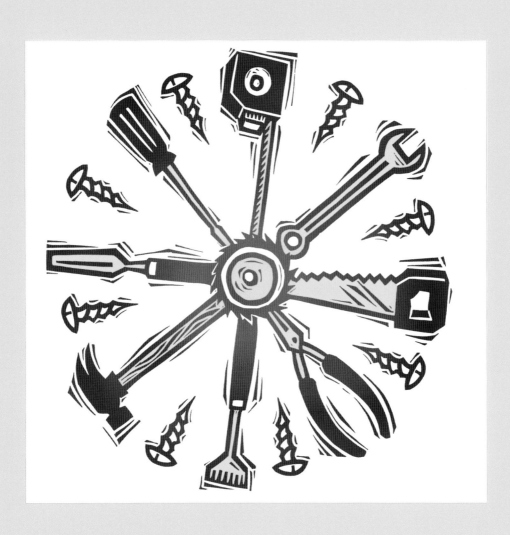

Home Maintenance

9

Running a home is an art, and the art of home maintenance has not always been given the respect it deserves. Usually, the work it takes to keep things running smoothly gets noticed only when something comes to a stop, breaks down or blows up. In this chapter, you can make notes on what it takes to keep your home in order.

There is room to document information on two homes, in case you have a vacation or other second home. List the people you would normally call for routine service and emergency repairs. Include contact information, means of delivery, account numbers, method of payment, and any other details you think useful. Note where owner manuals, warrantees and receipts can be found. Also specify anything in your home that isn't owned but is rented or leased; for instance, a water heater or office equipment.

Main residence

The property described here will be your primary residence. If you have more than one property, see also *Vacation home or other residence* at page 104.

Utilities

◆ electricity _____

◆ water _____

◆ telephone _____
_____

◆ oil/gas _____

◆ internet _____

Service/repair providers

- closest grocery store, bank, other conveniences _____

- painter _____
- plumber _____
- electrician _____
- general repair _____

- appliance service _____

- heating / air-conditioning _____

- lawn and garden care _____

- cleaning _____
- septic tank maintenance _____
- pool service _____
- snow removal _____

Do you have any maintenance contracts? (furnace plan, lawn care, automotive service, etc.)

For vehicles and motorized tools, see Chapter 10.

Garbage and recycling

- pickup _____
- closest garbage and recycling facility _____

Outdoors

Note any special care instructions and purchase, warranty and maintenance records or other information as might be needed.

- roof, eavestroughs, drain pipes

- gardens, plantings, lawn, compost

- landscaping, fences, walls

- in-ground or other watering system

- outdoor lighting solar equipment (heating, lights, panels)

- septic bed, weeping tiles, sump pump discharge, well

- screens, storm windows/doors, shutters, canopy, awnings

- deck, patio
- garden equipment, tools

- outdoor furniture
- barbecue, outdoor heater
- firewood
- greenhouse, garage/shed
- pool, hot tub, sauna, pond, fountain, other water features

- water safety (rescue equipment)

Security

- building, home security system, motion sensors

- smoke alarms (change batteries when the clock falls back or springs forward)

◆ fire extinguisher (location, expiry date) _____

_____

◆ home safe _____

◆ Who has keys to your home? (family, friends, neighbor, superintendant, landlord, cleaning service, painter, dog-walker, pool service, other?)

_____

_____

_____

◆ Who knows security passwords for your home?

_____

_____

Mail

◆ mailbox number _____

◆ home delivery _____

◆ post office box _____

Indoors

Note any special care instructions and purchase, warranty and maintenance records or other information as might be needed.

◆ electrical, generator _____

◆ lighting _____

◆ furnace, other heating _____

◆ air conditioning, fans _____

◆ water heater _____

◆ plumbing, drains, septic system, sump pump _____

◆ fireplace, wood stove _____

◆ central or other vacuum _____

- appliances _____

- wine cellar, cold storage _____

- whirlpool bath, special shower, other bathroom fixtures _____

- pest control _____
- cleaning and other maintenance _____

- tools, power tools, shop equipment, ladders, hardware (see also *Chapter 10, Vehicles and Motorized Tools*) _____

- filters, lightbulbs, batteries and other things that have to be replaced _____

- plants _____
- special care of furnishings _____

Where are they?

Gas, water and electric meters _____

Indoor shutoffs for water lines to outside _____

Main water line _____
Basement drain _____

Phone line in (test line) _____
Main electrical panel switch _____

Fuel (oil, propane) tank _____

Other _____

Vacation home or other residence

There may be some categories here that don't fit your vacation home. If, for instance, it's a one-room cabin deep in the woods, you likely don't have to worry about a security system or appliance repair. Don't forget to add local contacts to *Chapter 1, Important People.*

Utilities
(suppliers, means of delivery, account information, method of payment)

- electricity _____
- water / sewers _____
- telephone _____
- oil / gas _____
- internet _____

Service/repair providers

- painter _____
- plumber _____
- electrician _____
- general repair _____

- appliance service _____

- heating / air-conditioning _____
- lawn and garden care _____
- cleaning _____
- well-digging, septic tank maintenance _____

- water installation / winterizing _____

- snow removal _____

- tree-trimming / brush cutting _____

Do you have any maintenance contracts? (furnace plan, road clearing, pest control, seasonal security, etc.) _____

Garbage and recycling

◆ pickup _____

◆ compost _____

◆ closest garbage and recycling facility _____

_____

Outdoors

Note any special care instructions and purchase, warranty and maintenance records or other information as might be needed.

◆ roof, eavestroughs, drain pipes _____

◆ screens, storm windows / doors, shutters, canopy, awnings

_____

◆ driveway, fences, walls _____

◆ outdoor furniture _____

◆ outdoor lighting _____

◆ well, drinking water _____

◆ septic bed (note location of opening) _____

_____

◆ landscaping, gardens, lawn, compost _____

_____

◆ greenhouse, garden equipment, tools, garage / shed _____

_____

◆ barbecue, firepit, outdoor heating, firewood _____

_____

◆ pool, hot tub, sauna, pond, other water features _____

_____

◆ dock, raft _____

◆ boathouse _____

◆ water safety, rescue equipment _____

_____

◆ seasonal challenges _____

_____

For vehicles and motorized tools, see Chapter 10.

Security

- property, buildings
- home safe
- fire extinguisher, smoke alarms
- Who has keys to your home?

Mail

- mailbox number
- home delivery
- post office box

Indoors

Note any special care instructions and purchase, warranty and maintenance records or other information as might be needed.

- electrical, lighting

- furnace, fireplace, wood stove, other heating

- air conditioning, fans

- plumbing, drains, septic, sump pump

- appliances, water heater

- bathroom and kitchen fixtures

- pest control
- cleaning, other maintenance
- tools, power tools, shop equipment, ladders, hardware (see also *Chapter 10, Vehicles and Motorized Tools*)

- filters, lightbulbs, batteries and other things that have to be replaced

- special care of furnishings, plants, other

- winterizing

Where are they?

Gas, water and electric meters _____

Indoor shutoffs for water lines to outside _____

Main water line _____
Basement drain _____

Phone line in (test line) _____
Main electrical panel switch _____

Fuel (oil, propane) tank _____

Other _____

Extended Absence Checklist

If you regularly leave your home unoccupied for long periods of time you will undoubtedly have created a checklist of things to do to close up your home. You may have to redirect mail and cancel or suspend services such as phone, cable TV and newspaper delivery. If you have an alarm system, notify the security company of your absence and when you intend to return. They will ask for contact information for anyone who will be checking on your property. Consult with your home insurance agent to see what your policy requires.

My family's Thanksgiving weekend cottage closing chores include putting away boats, safeguarding plumbing against winter freezing and cleaning out all food and items attractive to mice. My mother's to-do list for closing up her winter home in Florida for the summer is more about leaving her place uninviting to mold, mildew and insects. She has someone come in regularly to spray for bugs and check that the thermostat and dehumidifier readings are okay.

Your list will vary depending on the kind of home and climate you live in. Note important chores and contact information here, tuck your checklist into the pocket at the back of this book, or indicate where it can be found.

_____

_____

_____

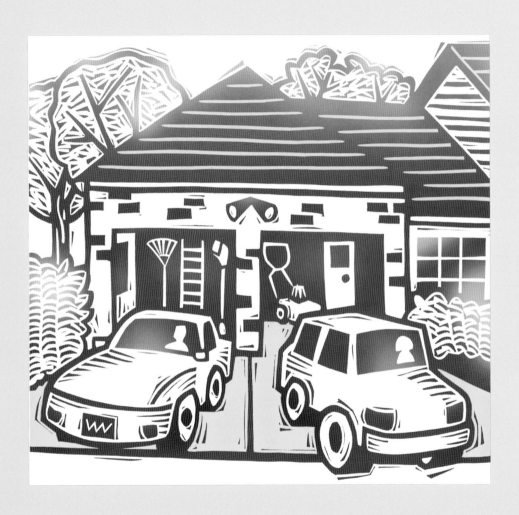

Vehicles and Motorized Tools

10

O pen your garage door and what do you see inside? The means to get around town — or out of it? Enough tools to start a hardware store? Many of us see a lot of expensive equipment in need of regular maintenance. Most modern households depend on one or more vehicles for basic transportation. And then there are the specialized vehicles some of us use for work, and the ones we use just for fun, such as all-terrain vehicles and snowmobiles. Your garage may also house a motorcycle, bicycles, even a treasured antique car. Your vacation property may include a shed that protects an ancient fishing boat or a grand boathouse that shelters a fleet of elegant watercraft. In addition to the vehicles you own, there are the motorized tools such as lawnmowers, trimmers and power washers.

Use this chapter to make notes on your cars, boats, bikes and other vehicles, as well the motorized tools that you use to maintain your property.

Vehicles

In this section, record information about any vehicles you own, lease or regularly use or store. Include contact information (especially for maintenance and insurance) and the location of important records.

Land vehicles

Include cars, minivans, SUVs and trucks; motorcycles and motorized bikes; trailers, campers and RVs; ATVs and snowmobiles; golf carts, mobility carts, scooters and wheelchairs; antique, show cars and other valuable vehicles.

For each of your vehicles, provide information where relevant about:
- name, model, brand, dealer, place of purchase
- VINs, ownership info, driver's /operator's licenses
- purchase, leasing or other agreements
- insurance (see also *Insurance* at page 92), assessed value

- parking, storage arrangements
- maintenance, service, repair records and providers
- any maintenance agreements, extended warranties
- fuel and other requirements, any tricks to operating
- tires, winter tires, chains
- trailer; other transport, towing or hauling equipment

Putting away your car for the winter

Yes, this is an activity known mostly to those who live in northern realms, particularly snowbirds who travel south for the winter and car enthusiasts who don't want to test their treasured vehicles in snow and icy conditions. What do the experts suggest if you are going to leave your car unused for a length of time?

- Change the oil before you put the car away.
- Fill the gas tank.
- Loosen and oil the spark plugs.
- Make sure tires are filled.
- Check your coolant antifreeze to make sure it is effective at expected temperatures.
- Clean the car, inside and out.

Charge and remove the battery. Do not place it on a concrete floor or near where anyone might be sleeping. Or else invest in a battery maintainer (a mechanical one) and have someone (your human battery maintainer) start the car every few weeks.

Bicycles

- name, model, brand, place of purchase
- storage, transport (bike rack), helmet, panniers and other gear
- maintenance
- insurance, warranty
- security identification, lock combination or keys

Boats and other watercraft

- ownership information, history, place of purchase
- insurance
- operator's license / permit
- docking or other storage arrangements
- maintenance, service agreements and records
- fuel and other requirements, operating tricks
- trailer, other transport or hauling equipment
- other boating and related sports equipment (water-skis, safety equipment, etc.)

Other power toys and garage gear

List and include instructions, warranty information, and any other relevant information for your lawnmower, snowblower, leafblower, power washer and any other power toys and gear you store in your garage here.

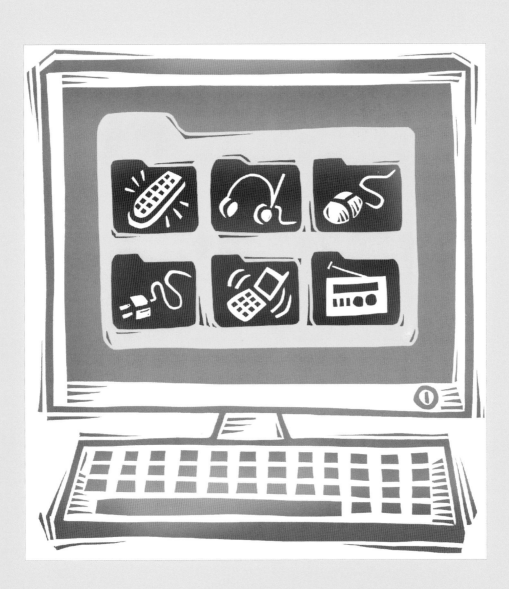

Computers, TVs and Other Technology

11

It happens to the best of us. You don't know how to record your favorite TV show, nor can you save your photographs to your computer and then send them to a friend. You haven't got a clue what made your computer crash, you can't remember your online banking PIN or the e-mail address your partner used to order virus protection software for the entire family. You don't know how to program the timer for the outside lights. You are ready to start throwing every little bit of electronic equipment you own out the window. Or maybe you are the tech head in your house, but your cohabitants are the clueless ones. Short of assigning your 12-year-old, card-carrying Geek Squad member nephew to active duty, what can you do?

Write it all down here. If you write down instructions, passwords, contact information and anything else you'll need to know to keep things working or to get help, you won't have to try to remember everything yourself. Nor will you have to worry about explaining everything to someone else if you have to go away or for some reason are not going to be able to help any more.

Computers

Provide all necessary details or note where they can be found.

◆ What kind of computer(s) do you have? What make, brand, model number? If there is a serial number, service tag or other number the manufacturer uses to identify your computer, record it here.

_____

_____

_____

_____

_____

◆ Where purchased?

◆ Where are receipts and warranty information?

◆ Are there any account numbers, user names or passwords necessary to operate the computer? What are they and or where are they kept?

◆ What kind of printers, scanners, or other peripheral equipment do you have? Give details as needed.

◆ Do you have separate hard drives, memory keys, cards or other storage devices?

◆ Do you use on-line or other off-site file storage?

◆ Where do you store important information and records? Photographs?

◆ What software programs do you have? Where are original disks / files / product keys / instructions for programs kept? If any of your software was downloaded, do you have the original download information?

◆ Are you on a network? Who else has access to it?

◆ Do you synchronize a cell phone, personal digital assistant (PDA) or other device with one or more of your computers? Are there any necessary pass-words or other codes?

◆ Is there anything on your computer you would like deleted before anyone else is allowed to use it?

◆ Who supplies your internet service? How do you pay for it?

◆ What are the settings needed to access your internet? _____

◆ What are your e-mail addresses? What are they used for? How can the mail be accessed if necessary? _____

◆ Do you belong to Facebook or any other social networking sites?

◆ What online services or subscriptions (such as an antivirus program, online journal or game system) do you subscribe to? _____

◆ How do you pay for these services and subscriptions? _____

◆ What other services do you access through the internet? (See also *Chapter 7, Finance*). Online banking? bill paying? file storage? _____

◆ Is there any essential information (documents, records, photographs, for instance) on your computer that must be saved? Where can it be found?

◆ Is there anyone else who knows how to operate your computer(s) and other technology? _____

◆ Have you ever had any of this equipment serviced? By whom? Would you call them again or recommend someone else? _____

◆ Are there any special tricks to operating your computer or related equipment?

Cameras and other photographic equipment; photos and videos

Note details about any photographic equipment or gear you own including description, serial numbers if you have them, place of purchase, warranties, location of equipment, receipts and manuals, where you go to have your equipment serviced and the location of any other useful information.

◆ Do you send files out to be printed or film out to be developed? What film lab / developing / print service do you use?

◆ How do you store your photos, slides, videos? Where can they be found?

TV and sound and other entertainment systems

◆ What equipment do you have?

◆ Where purchased? Do you have receipts, warranties? Where?

◆ Do you subscribe to any cable, satellite or other services? Who supplies them and how do you pay?

◆ Are there any account numbers, user names or passwords associated with these systems or services?

◈ Have you had equipment serviced? Wiring installed? By whom? Would you call them again?

◈ Are there any tricks to operating this equipment?

◈ Where do you keep the remote controls? How do you turn the TV on?

(For music collections and video collections, see *Chapter 12, Favorite Things*.)

Other electronics

Describe items and note where they were purchased and where they are kept. Detail receipts, warranties and manuals; any accounts, contracts, subscriptions or service providers; special features, memory cards or keys; and any other information necessary to operation (including phone numbers, passwords and identification).

Cell phone, PDA (includes Blackberry, Palm Pilot, iPhone or other)

MP3 players, iPods, personal sound systems

Intercoms, walkie talkies, CB radio, ham radio

Game systems, GPS devices and other electronics

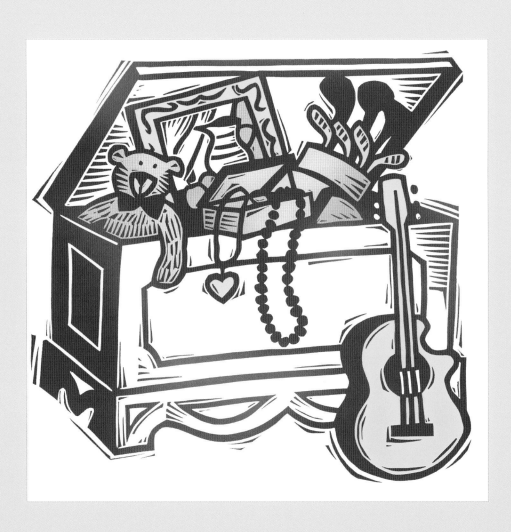

Your Favorite Things

12

In this chapter you can make notes on the location, care, maintenance, history and worth of your favorite things and valuables. Of course, your favorite things won't necessarily be of great monetary value nor the same things family members and friends value. Your most precious objects may be important to you because of the memories they hold and events or people they represent.

That point aside, it is hard for some of us to know what is valuable in the money sense and what is not. Have you had your valuables appraised? Have you done a photographic inventory? If you do have an inventory and appraisals, those records are important, and not just for insurance or for your heirs. The information is also useful for anyone who might have to take care of your things if you cannot.

By making notes in this chapter, you can create a record for yourself and at the same time provide information for others. If there are particular objects you want to be looked after, or that need special servicing, you can give directions for care. Additionally, should you choose to ask someone to sell objects for you — if, for instance, you are moving — you will already have a record of what you started out with.

You may wish to also note if there is anything specific you want to bequeath to anyone, though bequests are best written into your will.

Inventory

Some people inventory their belongings, noting serial numbers, date and place of purchase, and identifying items with descriptions and in photographs. If you have, note where the record of your inventory can be found.

Art

Antiques

Jewelry

China, crystal and silver

Wine, cigars, other consumables

Furnishings

Collections, rarities

Sentimental favorites

Pianos and other musical instruments

Arts and crafts supplies, tools

Clothing

Books, music, videos

Photographs

Sports and recreation equipment

Guns, weapons

Awards, trophies, mementos

Other

Do you have any secret hiding places for your treasures?

Many people have a "secret hiding place" in which they hide cash, jewelry, guns, ammunition, liquor, love letters or some other personal treasure. Make sure that the right people know if you have any special hiding places!

Collectors

If you are planning to leave anything — art, historical artifacts or photographs, for instance — to a gallery, museum or historical society, you should first check if they want it. Have the value assessed, tell them after you have made up your will, and follow up with a letter of intent.

Are you a borrower or a lender?

Have any valuable items been lent out to friends or relatives with the intention that they are to be returned to you? Have any items been given to friends or family with "no strings attached"? Have you borrowed anything from anyone — with the understanding that you will return it to them? Provide details.

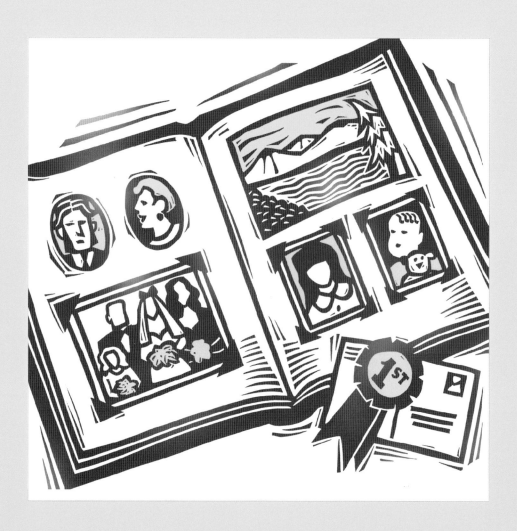

Personal History

13

Your own personal history is worth writing down. You are an individual and you have your own story entirely distinct from anyone else's. Genealogists know the thrill of tracking down that one individual who forms the link between two seemingly unconnected people years and years ago. We are all connected one way or another. Your story is worth something to you and to someone else — your family, your friends, a neighbor, someone — even if you don't know who that someone else is right now. Write it down!

About me

Record relevant dates and places and the people involved — give details.

Birth

Religious and spiritual rites (baptism, bar mitzvah, other)

Marriage

Divorce / Separation

Children

Adoption

Foster parents, children

Other dependents

Education history

Employment history

Volunteer service

Military service

Travel history

Special skills and accomplishments

Other

Your family tree

Fill in the names, occupations, dates and places of birth, baptism, marriage, residence, military service, death and other information with as much or as little detail as you wish. Use the categories given here or make up your own to suit your family circumstances. Make future genealogists happy!

Mother

Father

Maternal grandparents

Paternal grandparents

Siblings

Spouse/partner(s)

Children

Grandchildren

In-laws: spouse/partners' parents and siblings

Aunts, uncles, cousins, nieces, nephews

Other family members

Where are they now?

Do you know where your ancestors are buried? Who has the deeds for the burial plots of your ancestors and other relatives?

To record your family medical history, see *Chapter 4, Health and Medical Care*.

Family documents
Where do you keep certificates or legal documents to mark births, deaths, adoptions, custody, baptismal or other religious rites, marriage, separation, divorce, prenuptial or postnuptial agreements?

Dates to remember

Note any family birthdates, anniversaries, holidays and other occasions you want
to be reminded of here.

DATE   PERSON / OCCASION / NOTES

_____   _____

_____   _____

_____   _____

_____   _____

_____   _____

_____   _____

_____   _____

_____   _____

_____   _____

_____   _____

_____   _____

_____   _____

_____   _____

Family treasures and traditions

Family recipes, holiday customs, family stories.... These are some of the things
that distinguish one family from another and make up the history of a person.
Share yours here.

_____

_____

_____

_____

_____

_____

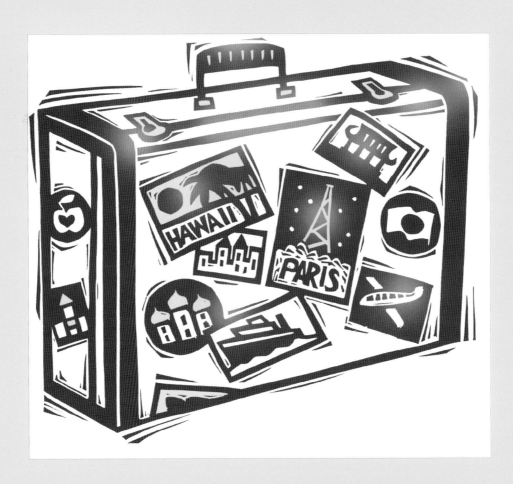

So Far Away

14

If you have ever been away from home for more than a few days, you know that things at home don't just take care of themselves. Perhaps you are away a lot or for long stretches of time. Perhaps you are in military service and posted across the country or the ocean. You or your partner may be working on an oil rig, doing time in prison, traveling for work or just like to stay late at the office a lot. You may be in a long-distance relationship, so you regularly spend weekends with your partner elsewhere. Or you have a medical condition that means you must leave your home for long-term care elsewhere. Perhaps you are a professor on a sabbatical and your family is doing a home exchange. Or you are a Snowbird, traveling south for the winter as soon as the snow begins to fly.

A lot of questions will arise in thinking about and planning for recurring or longer absences — yours or your partner's. The few that follow are just a sampling.

What should be done about…
- forwarding mail?
- paying bills?
- maintaining home and property?
- emergencies?
- powers of attorney, in case decisions such as selling property have to be made?

Other questions may seem minor, but knowing the answers can mean avoiding headaches:
- Where do you take the dry cleaning? Photos to be processed?
- Have you cancelled newspaper or other subscriptions?
- If you are a frequent traveler, where do you park your car at the airport? What is the make, model and license plate number?

Big-picture questions and matters of the heart will also arise:
- How will you keep in touch? Do LDRs (long-distance relationships) work?
- What are your favorite things? A "care package" might contain these.
- How are children or other dependents protected?

You will find space to answer these and many similar questions in other chapters in this book, but this chapter especially provides some thoughts about and space for subjects that relate particularly to long or recurring absences.

Military families

Military families have to deal with many stresses. Various organizations and support groups within and outside the military establishment offer advice on how families can best prepare for common stressful scenarios such as deployment, leaving, coming home, possible injury and death.

In the US, the national Military Family Association (www.nmfa.org) offers support and information on all kinds of matters, from communicating with your "service member" and tips on sending care packages, to practical preparations for deployment, including child-care backup planning.

Canadian Forces members and their families can turn to the CF Family Resources website (www.forces.gc.ca/site/fam/index-eng.asp) for information about military life, support services and programs and links to support groups such as Canadian Forces Wives and Girlfriends. In the United Kingdom, the Ministry of Defence offers links, information and guidance for members of the Service community through its website: www.mod.uk/DefenceInternet/DefenceFor/ServiceCommunity/.

Families of inmates

In March 2009 the *San Francisco Sentinel* reported, based on a Pew Center on the States study in 2007, that "The U.S. correctional population — those in jail, prison, on probation or on parole — totaled 7.3 million, or 1 in every 31 adults."

If you have the misfortune to find yourself an inmate or have a partner in prison, do whatever you can to avail yourself of the available resources. For example, Prison Fellowship is a faith-based charity that helps prison inmates and their families with summer camps, pen-pal programs and other services. One program they run is called Angel Tree: volunteers collect donations and give their own time to ensure that children of inmates will have something from their parent waiting for them under the tree at Christmas.

On the road again

What do truckers, offshore oil-rig operators, sales reps, movie stars, musicians and professional athletes have in common? A lot of time spent away from home — sometimes most of the year.

Most long-distance truck drivers are away from home all week long; some are gone for months at a time. Many jobs in mining, logging, fishing and other resource industries take workers away from home for long periods of time. Some sales representatives have large territories and must travel away from home for several days or weeks at a time. Similarly, professional musicians, actors and athletes and travel to perform, train or play.

If you or your partner has a job that requires travel or separation for long periods of time, how do you manage? The list that follows contains additional points to consider and perhaps discuss. You can make notes below.

- ways to keep in touch
- care packages, mail
- visits, travel leave
- having an emergency plan and updating it regularly
- banking, insurance and other financial arrangements
- making sure health and other benefits are continued
- creating powers of attorney
- child care and education
- naming guardians for dependents
- pets, plants and perishables
- closing up a home for months at a time
- putting away cars, boats for the season
- the pros and cons of renting versus owning
- making friends and finding your way in new places
- finding resources and support groups

Your Notes

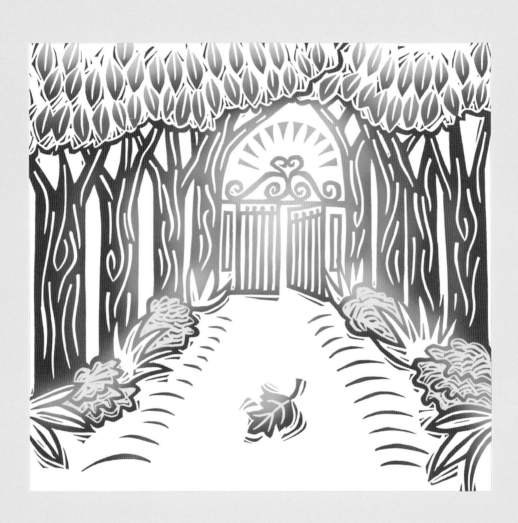

And in the End

15

There comes a time when you should think about your own death. Very few people want to think about dying, but here you have the opportunity to think and write about your wishes without anyone else answering for you. You can think about what you might want your end of life to be like, and any special medical wishes or advance directives you want to make known to those who might have to represent you if you are unable to speak for yourself. You can also prepare yourself and loved ones for your death by making your wishes known about such practical aspects as who to notify in the event of your death and where your important papers are. You can note what you want to be done with your body, if you want a funeral, memorial service or other ceremonial marking of your passing, and even what you want your obituary to say. You can be as specific or as general as you choose.

It is a lot easier to think about the end of your life when the events in question are not imminent and your good judgment is not clouded by fear or uncertainty. Do it now, knowing that you may change your mind when the time comes, but at least you have expressed your opinions today.

End of life and palliative care

Record any special wishes you have for your own medical and personal care as you approach the end of your life. You may find that some of your answers change as time goes by. You can always change your notes or otherwise indicate you have different wishes at the time.

What do you want in treatment in hospital?

What you want in treatment at home?

What are your thoughts on nursing homes and other care facilities?

Who should be notified if you know you don't have long to live?

Who can make health care and medical decisions for you? Have you created a power of attorney for health care? If you have not already provided contact information for your representative(s), turn to page 58.

Is there anyone you would like to visit with you? Anyone you would prefer not to see?

Do you have any food likes or dislikes? Do you like any special flowers?

Do you have any favorite clothing? Other comfort items? What are your favorite ways to keep warm or stay cool?

What is your favorite entertainment? Your favorite music, videos, books, card games or other?

Are there any special mementoes you would like to have with you if you have to move into a care facility? (Keep in mind, however, that many facilities discourage residents from having anything valuable for fear of theft or loss.)

Are there any activities you would like to continue when in care, if you are able to do so?

To what lengths and by what means you want medical care to keep you alive? (See also *Chapter 4, Health and Medical Care.*)

Preparing for death

Is there anything you would like to do before you die? Is there any "unfinished business" you want to attend to? Anyone you want to do anything special for? Are there any borrowed objects you want to return or debts you want to repay? Is there any person you want to see, any place you want to visit? Do you have any last wishes? Provide details and contact information as needed.

Do you have all your papers and legal documents in order? Do you have an up-to-date will? Is information about your will recorded in this book?

Are there financial arrangements you want to make before you die? Are there bank or investment accounts you would like to make into joint accounts with your heirs? Any trust funds you would like to set up? Any gifts you want to make? Have you sought the advice of a lawyer, accountant or estate advisor?

Do you have any religious or spiritual requests? Do you wish to see a member of the clergy or other spiritual advisor? Do you want to receive any sacraments or have any other blessings or rites performed while you are still alive?

Have you considered making and prepaying for your own funeral arrangements?

Have you written letters to family members to be opened when you die? Do they know where they are?

When I'm gone

There is no right or wrong way to prepare your family for your death, except perhaps to entirely ignore the prospect. Some people who are faced with a future of not living to see their children grow up prepare letters, video messages and gifts for when their kids are older. Some write out or tape a family history, or mark up photo albums with names and information, so the mystery people and places will have stories to go with them. Others crochet baby blankets or make quilts. Some get busy putting their estates and lives in order; some clean house. Some look for new mates for their partners in the hope that their children will have another parent to take their place. And some simply spend as much time as they can with their families when they are able to.

Organ donation

Have you signed your organ donor card? Where do you keep it? What are your wishes? Have you let your family and doctor know?

Life after death

Quite a number of decisions have to be made almost immediately after someone dies. Although historically our cultural customs and religious beliefs have dictated certain ceremonies and rituals after a death, more and more, personal preferences dictate what we do when it comes to laying our dead to rest.

You can help your survivors make decisions and ensure that your wishes are respected by indicating your choices and preferences here.

It may seem morbid to plan your own funeral, but it's actually a good idea to discuss your plans in advance with family and any close friends who may be involved in carrying out your wishes. Over the next few pages you can describe any arrangements you have already made, your wishes, the location of any relevant documents, and who to contact. Some choices that appear here may apply to you and others will not; use the space as best fits your purposes.

TIP: Funeral and burial plans should be readily accessible to your survivors. They should be in a document separate from the will, as the will is not usually read until days after the death. The only copy should not be in your safe deposit box either, as it is often sealed after death.

Notification

Who should be notified when you die? Is contact information noted in *Chapter 1, Important People*? If not, provide it here. If there is not enough room, you can attach a list or indicate where one can be found.

_____

_____

_____

Death notice or obituary: content, choice of newspapers, other publications

_____

_____

_____

_____

IT'S YOUR FUNERAL

Funeral home _____

_____

_____

_____

Wake, shiva, blessing, visitation with the family, other ceremony before the funeral _____

_____

_____

_____

Open or closed casket for visitation _____

Funeral ceremony, memorial or other _____

_____

Public or private ceremony _____

_____

Religious or other spiritual ceremony, place of worship

Clergy, other officiants, readers, speakers, eulogist

Favorite readings, poems, other

Favorite music, hymns

Suggested pallbearers

Casket

Chosen clothing, jewelry, other for body / mementoes to be placed with body

Burial

Cemetery, memorial garden, burial plot, other

Headstone or monument

Post-funeral reception

Cremation / cremation service

Disposition, special location of cremated remains

Memorial

Family or other customs

Remember me

Your survivors may choose to remember you with a donation to your favorite charity. Some people create teams for a run to raise money for medical research. Others sponsor a bench at a golfer's favorite course. Some remember a loved one with a newly planted tree at a favorite park or a stained-glass window at their place of worship. Someone could commemorate you by contributing to equipment for a local hospital or setting up a fund for a memorial scholarship. If you have a desire to be remembered in a particular way, find out if what you want is possible and make your wishes known here.

Your choice

Funerals and memorial services and ceremonies can vary in location, style, size and form. Some people find comfort in familiar rituals and some prefer to devise their own unique good-byes. Yours can be almost anything you choose:

- traditional
- religious
- humanist
- with singing or without
- with a eulogy or without
- eco-conscious, green
- long or short
- elaborate or "the Simple Alternative"
- in a church, synagogue, temple, mosque
- in a funeral home chapel
- in a funeral home, with a big-screen TV for a slide show and video
- in a church hall
- at a Legion Hall, with military honors
- at the cemetery
- at a memorial park
- at a pub
- at home, in your back yard
- at a school
- at an airshow
- at sea
- at the cottage

After-death checklist

If you are a recently bereaved next of kin and or the executor of a new estate, there are many things you will have to take on in the days after a death. This checklist covers some of the challenges. The names of the officials and organizations may be different in your location, but the tasks are generally the same. Be sure to take the advice of a funeral director — they do know what they are doing!

☐ After the death, call the person's doctor. If a doctor or emergency services are not available, or you are concerned about the circumstances of the death, contact your local coroner's office. If you know that organs or the body are to be donated, notify the next of kin (if that is not you) and the doctor. The doctor or coroner will complete a Medical Certificate of Death and give it to the funeral director to go with the body.

☐ Contact a funeral home or other transfer service. A family member and the funeral director together have to complete a Statement of Death (or Formal Notice). The funeral director will submit the certificate and statement to the municipal clerk's office to register the death. Depending on where you live, you or the funeral director may have to apply for permission for a burial or cremation.

☐ If not already done by the doctor or funeral home, apply for a death certificate. It will be needed for settling the estate, insurance purposes, access to accounts, government services, pensions and more. Get at least six copies to start.

☐ Contact people who need to be notified, relatives and close friends first.

☐ Arrange for care of children and adult dependents, if necessary.

☐ Arrange for care of pets.

☐ Keep a phone log at the house to record calls.

☐ Create to-do lists and cross off tasks as they are done.

☐ Look for any instructions the person may have left about funeral arrangements. Locate other important papers such as a will, birth and marriage certificates, social insurance/security cards and so on.

☐ Meet with the funeral director and prepare a death notice or obituary. If planning a religious funeral, call your church, synagogue or other place of worship to arrange possible times for a service. If you are sitting shiva, decide for how many days.

☐ Work with family members, funeral director and clergy or other involved parties to plan the funeral, memorial or other service or ceremony and the burial or cremation.

☐ Ask about how much the funeral and burial or cremation will cost. Unless the bill has been prepaid, you may end up paying, at least until the estate is settled. Some pension and veteran's plans and insurance will pay a lump sum to help with funeral costs.

☐ Cancel home deliveries. Make sure the person's residence is safe and secured. Make sure someone is at the house during the funeral to foil burglars who read death notices.

☐ Make sure you have authority to deal with the estate. Contact a lawyer or other legal advisor if there is no will. If you are executor of the estate, see duties of an executor at page 37 in *Chapter 3, Legal Advice*. You will be in charge of distributing the estate to the beneficiaries paying off debts, including funeral expenses, filing a final tax return, and many of the other tasks listed below. You will be entitled to receive fair compensation for your time and effort.

☐ Contact banks, credit card companies, lending and other financial institutions. Cancel direct debits and deposits.

☐ Locate safe deposit box.

☐ Contact former employers. Investigate employee benefits and union benefits.

☐ Contact life insurance, property and automobile insurance companies.

☐ Contact government offices, including tax / revenue departments, and any that might distribute or cancel benefits (for old age pension, disability, veteran's funerals, bereavement or survivor's benefits, savings bonds, guardian's allowance, child tax credits, etc.).

☐ Apply for benefits where entitled: check time limits for application.

☐ Look into car ownership and license, real estate and property deeds, property taxes; cable TV, telephone, electric and other utility companies.

☐ Cancel subscriptions, redirect mail.

☐ Advise the person's doctors, dentist, employers, social services, schools, alumni associations, professional, business and other contacts.

☐ Return library books and any other borrowed items. Claim refunds on season's tickets, club memberships, union dues.

◆ Accept offers of help where you can. Most people don't know what to do for the newly bereaved, so don't hesitate to be direct and make specific requests.

◆ Look after yourself, physically and emotionally. Surround yourself with people who are good for you and avoid those who are not. Find someone you trust to listen when you need to talk things over.

Acknowledgments

I offer my gratitude to all who have helped me in the writing and putting together of this book. Thanks to those at Firefly Books who have helped shepherd it along. Thank you to Noel Hudson and John Denison for friendship, encouragement, advice and adventures through our years together as Boston Mills Press. Thank you to artist Sue Todd, for your beautiful work and your patience — I'm so glad I found you! Thank you to friend, designer and BMP style-setter Gill Stead for taking this idea and making it look good — the book and the getting there wouldn't have been nearly as fine without you.

Special thanks to friends and family who offered their own experiences as fodder for this book and listened when I went on and on about pet funerals and powers of attorney.

With love to my next of kin, and in memory of dear ones already gone...

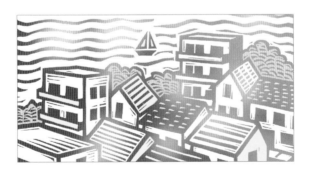

Selected Reading

Included here are a number of the books that have been of use to me in the writing of this book. It is by no means an exhaustive list of all the resources available. Visit your local bookstore or library and seek out these and other sources of information, and consult professionals, individuals and associations knowledgeable in the subjects you want to learn about.

Blacklock, Jean, Myashiro, Judy and Susan Murphy. *Food for Thought: Bringing Estate Planning to Life*. Toronto: John Wiley & Sons Canada, Ltd., 2001.

Callanan, Maggie and Patricia Kelley. *Final Gifts: Understanding the Special Awareness, Needs and Communications of the Dying*. New York, NY: Bantam Dell, 1992.

Cardy, Sandy with Michael Fitzgerald. *The Cottage, the Spider Brooch, and the Second Wife: How to Overcome the Challenges of Estate Planning*. Toronto: ECW Press, 2003.

Edenfield, Ann. *Family Arrested: How to Survive the Incarceration of a Loved One*. Albuquerque, NM: Americana Publishing, Inc. 2002.

Ellis, Deborah. *Off to War: Voices of Soldiers' Children*. Toronto, ON / Berkeley, CA: Groundwood Books, 2008.

Foster, Sandra E. *You Can't Take It With You: Common-Sense Estate Planning for Canadians*. Fifth Edition. Mississauga, ON: John Wiley & Sons Canada, Ltd., 2007.

Henderson, Kristin. *While They're at War: The True Story of American Families on the Homefront*. New York, NY: Houghton Mifflin Company, 2006.

Hunter, Douglas. *The Cottage Ownership Guide: How to Buy, Sell, Rent, Share, Hand Down & Retire to Your Waterfront Getaway*. Toronto/Buffalo: Cottage Life Books, 2006.

Kellehear, Allan. *A Social History of Dying*. New York: Cambridge University Press, 2007.

Kiernan, Stephen P. *Last Rights: Rescuing the End of Life from the Medical System*. New York: St. Martin's Press, 2006.

Kubler-Ross, Elisabeth. *On Death and Dying: What the dying have to teach doctors, nurses, clergy, and their own families*. New York, NY: MacMillan 1969, Scribner 2003.

Ross, Judy Smith. *Good Grief, I Have to Plan a Funeral: A Detailed Guide to Planning a Funeral*. Thornbury, Ontario: Valley Girls Publishing, 2004.

Self-Counsel Press offers many publications of interest to American and Canadian readers.

Schiff, Harriet Sarnoff. *The Bereaved Parent*. Toronto: Penguin Books, 1981.

Simpson, Sheila. *The Survivor's Guide: Coping with the Details of Death*. Toronto: Summerhill Press, 1990.

Wylie, Betty Jane. *Life's Losses: Living Through Grief, Bereavement, and Sudden Change*. Toronto: Macmillan Press, 1996.

Index